LOW CARB HIGH PROTEIN COOKBOOK

150 Tasty, Quick, Low-Carb Dishes to Shed Pounds and Strengthen Muscles in Just 28 Days. Includes 60-Day Meal Plan

CRESSIDA LANE

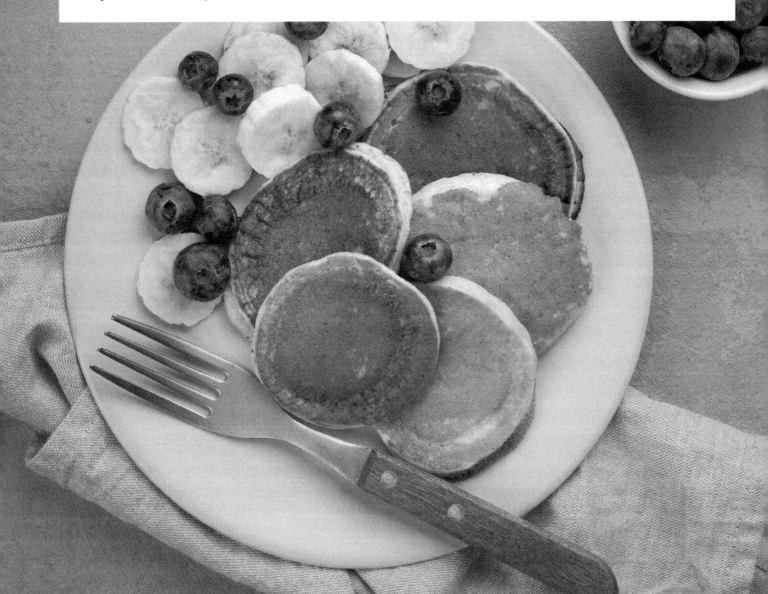

Table of Contents

CHAPTER 4
HEALTHY AND FAST LUNCHES

CHAPTER 5
FAMILY-FRIENDLY DINNERS

CHAPTER 8
YOUR 28-DAY JUMPSTART: THE FIRST FOUR WEEKS

CHAPTER 9
THE COMPLETE 60-DAY MEAL PLAN: SUSTAINABLE RESULTS

CHAPTER 10
HOW TO CALCULATE AND ADJUST YOUR CALORIC NEEDS

CHAPTER 11
EASY SUBSTITUTIONS: ADAPTING RECIPES TO FIT YOUR LIFESTYLE

Introduction

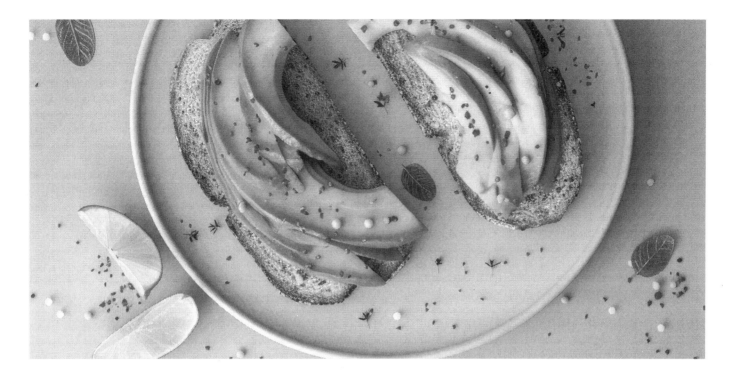

Imagine a way of eating that leaves you feeling full, energized, and fit without the constant hunger pangs, energy crashes, or endless hours spent meal prepping. Welcome to the **Low Carb, High Protein lifestyle**, a balanced and sustainable approach to healthy eating that focuses on nourishing your body while helping you achieve your goals of weight loss, muscle toning, and overall wellness. This isn't just another fad diet that will leave you feeling frustrated or overwhelmed. It's a flexible way of eating that can easily adapt to your life, no matter how busy or chaotic it gets.

The idea of low-carb eating has been around for a while, and for good reason. Cutting back on carbohydrates and increasing protein intake can have transformative effects on your body. Carbohydrates, especially those found in processed and refined foods, can often lead to energy spikes and crashes, leaving you feeling drained and struggling to manage your appetite. By contrast, protein provides a steady source of energy, keeps you feeling fuller for longer, and supports muscle growth and repair—essential if your goal is to tone up or maintain lean muscle while losing fat.

However, the Low Carb, High Protein lifestyle isn't just about cutting out carbs entirely or depriving yourself of the foods you love. It's about balance and making smarter choices that fit into your day-to-day life. This book is designed to help you make those choices without feeling like you're constantly making sacrifices. You don't need to feel restricted or miss out on family dinners, social events, or the enjoyment of a good meal. Instead, you'll learn how to make simple adjustments to your diet that allow you to eat delicious, satisfying meals that also help you meet your health and fitness goals.

One of the biggest challenges when it comes to changing your eating habits is how overwhelming it can feel. If you've ever tried a diet before, you've probably experienced the frustration of following a plan that's complicated, time-consuming, and unsustainable. You might have found yourself spending hours in the kitchen preparing meals that don't taste as good as you'd hoped, or worse, giving up because it was too hard to stick to the plan. The Low Carb, High Protein approach is different. It's built for real life, with recipes that are quick and easy to prepare, ingredients that are simple to find, and meal plans that are flexible enough to fit around your busy schedule.

This way of eating is particularly well-suited to people like you—busy professionals, parents, and anyone who has a lot on their plate. Life is hectic enough without having to worry about complicated meal prep or trying to figure out whether you're eating the "right" foods. In this book, you'll find meals that are designed to be quick to prepare, family-friendly, and most importantly, full of flavor. You'll discover how to whip up meals in under 30 minutes that your whole family will love, whether you're making a breakfast omelet packed with veggies, a quick chicken salad for lunch, or a hearty, protein-rich dinner that keeps everyone satisfied.

But this book isn't just a collection of recipes. It's a roadmap to a healthier lifestyle that goes beyond the food you eat. You'll learn how to make meal planning easy, how to stay motivated when life gets hectic, and how to set realistic goals for your health and fitness. This is not about reaching a certain number on the scale or following a rigid set of rules—it's about feeling stronger, more energetic, and more in control of your health. By focusing on nutrient-dense, high-protein foods, you'll be fueling your body with the right kind of energy that supports your busy lifestyle, whether that means managing a demanding job, keeping up with your kids, or simply wanting to feel your best every day.

The Low Carb, High Protein lifestyle isn't about perfection. It's about progress and finding a balance that works for you. One of the key principles behind this way of eating is sustainability. You don't need to give up entire food groups, nor do you need to be constantly counting calories or obsessing over what you eat. Instead, you'll focus on eating more of the foods that fuel your body properly—lean proteins, healthy fats, and nutrient-dense vegetables—while cutting back on processed carbs and sugars that offer little nutritional value.

For many people, the hardest part of starting a new diet is dealing with cravings and feeling deprived. We've all been there—trying to resist that piece of bread or chocolate bar, only to give in and feel guilty later. The good news is, with the Low Carb, High Protein approach, you don't have to feel like you're depriving yourself. In fact, many of the meals in this book are designed to be indulgent while still supporting your health goals. Think creamy avocado and salmon toast for breakfast, a satisfying steak salad for lunch, or a delicious bowl of zucchini noodles with pesto and chicken for dinner. You'll also find plenty of guilt-free desserts and snacks, so you can enjoy treats like chocolate protein pudding or peanut butter cups without feeling like you've strayed from your plan.

In addition to delicious recipes, this book also includes flexible meal plans that are easy to follow and designed to help you stay on track. Whether you're looking for a 28-day jumpstart to kick off your health journey or a more long-term 60-day meal plan to sustain your progress, you'll find everything you need here. These plans are built with real life in mind—no complicated shopping lists or hours of meal prep required. You'll learn how to prep ingredients in advance, make smart swaps to suit your preferences, and adapt the plans to fit your specific goals, whether that's losing weight, building muscle, or simply maintaining a healthy lifestyle.

Most importantly, this book will show you that healthy eating doesn't have to be hard. It doesn't have to be complicated, restrictive, or time-consuming. With the right guidance, a few simple changes, and delicious, easy-to-prepare meals, you can transform the way you eat and feel better than ever. By the time you reach the end of this book, you'll have the tools and knowledge you need to create lasting, positive changes in your life—without giving up the foods you love or sacrificing precious time with your family.

So, whether you're here to lose weight, gain more energy, or simply find a more sustainable way of eating that fits into your busy life, you've come to the right place. This journey is about more than just the food you eat. It's about finding balance, achieving your goals, and feeling empowered to take control of your health. The Low Carb, High Protein lifestyle is here to support you every step of the way. Welcome to your new way of eating, living, and thriving.

CHAPTER 1

Welcome to the Low Carb, High Protein Lifestyle

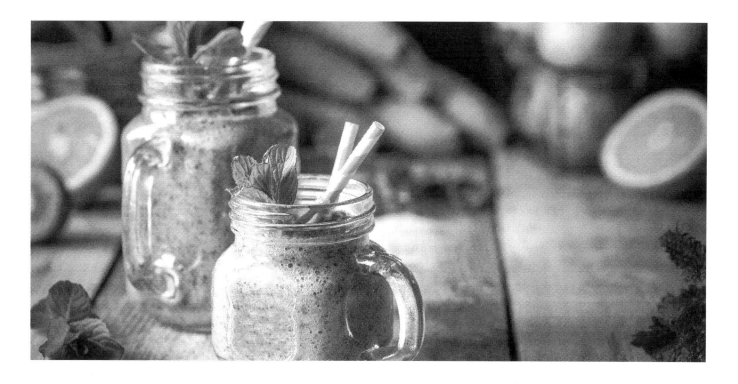

Life is a delicate balance between what we need to do and what we want to do. In our fast-paced modern world, this balancing act becomes even more challenging. Between work, family, social commitments, and personal aspirations, it's easy for self-care—particularly our diet and nutrition—to slip through the cracks. Most of us have been there, juggling one too many things and grabbing the quickest meal we can find, whether or not it fuels our bodies properly. That's where the **Low Carb, High Protein lifestyle** comes in: an approach to eating that is not just a temporary fix but a sustainable, long-term solution designed to fit into your busy life while delivering the results you've been seeking. This isn't a trend or a diet fad—it's a way of nourishing your body that empowers you to take control of your health without feeling restricted or deprived.

Why This Diet Works

When you hear the phrase "low-carb," you might immediately think of cutting out bread, pasta, and all the indulgent carbs you've come to love. But this lifestyle is much more nuanced than simply slashing carbs. The key to the **Low Carb, High Protein** diet is understanding how our bodies process different types of macronutrients—carbohydrates, proteins, and fats—and using this knowledge to make more balanced food choices that help our bodies function at their best.

At its core, the Low Carb, High Protein approach works by focusing on reducing the consumption of carbohydrates—particularly refined and processed ones—while increasing the intake of lean proteins and healthy fats. Carbohydrates, especially simple ones like sugars and refined grains, are quickly broken down into glucose in the bloodstream, causing blood sugar spikes. These spikes are followed by crashes that leave us feeling tired, irritable, and craving more quick energy, often in the form of more carbs. It's a cycle that many people are stuck in, leading to energy highs and lows throughout the day.

By reducing your carb intake, particularly those fast-digesting carbs, and replacing them with protein and healthy fats, you create a more stable energy flow throughout the day. Protein plays a crucial role in this process. Unlike carbohydrates, protein takes longer for the body to break down, which helps keep you feeling full and satisfied for longer. It also has a much lower impact on blood sugar, preventing those energy crashes that leave you feeling depleted. Protein also helps build and repair muscle, making it essential for anyone looking to tone up or maintain muscle mass while losing fat.

But the beauty of the Low Carb, High Protein lifestyle is that it's not just about reducing carbohydrates for the sake of cutting something out. It's about focusing on **quality**—choosing whole, nutrient-dense foods that nourish your body and provide sustained energy. By prioritizing protein, you're giving your body the fuel it needs to build and repair tissues, support metabolic function, and keep you feeling strong and energized. And by being more mindful about the types of carbohydrates you consume—choosing complex, fiber-rich options like vegetables and whole grains—you're ensuring that your body has the essential nutrients it needs without overloading it with unnecessary sugars.

What makes this approach so effective for weight loss and muscle maintenance is its ability to help you burn fat while preserving lean muscle mass. When you reduce your carb intake, your body begins to rely more on stored fat for energy, which can help accelerate fat loss. At the same time, increasing protein intake helps protect your muscle mass, ensuring that the weight you lose is primarily fat, not muscle. This is crucial for maintaining a toned, fit appearance and for keeping your metabolism functioning optimally.

Moreover, a **Low Carb, High Protein** diet can also have positive effects on other aspects of health. Studies have shown that it can improve blood sugar control, reduce cholesterol levels, and support cardiovascular health. It's also been linked to improvements in mental clarity and focus, as stabilizing your blood sugar helps prevent the brain fog that can come from energy crashes.

For many, the most immediate benefit of adopting a Low Carb, High Protein lifestyle is the reduction in cravings and hunger pangs. Because protein and fat are more satiating than car-bohydrates, you're likely to feel fuller for longer, which helps prevent overeating and snacking on unhealthy foods. It's a way of eating that doesn't feel like deprivation, and that's what makes it so sustainable. You're not constantly battling hunger or feeling like you're missing out on your favorite foods. Instead, you're enjoying meals that are both delicious and nutritious, helping you stay on track with your health goals without feeling like you're on a "diet."

How This Book Can Change Your Life

You're probably reading this book because you're ready for a change. Maybe you've tried other diets before, only to feel frustrated when they didn't deliver the lasting results you were hoping for. Maybe you're tired of feeling sluggish, constantly battling cravings, or struggling to find the time to prepare healthy meals amidst the chaos of daily life. Whatever your reasons, this book is here to provide you with a solution—a roadmap to a healthier, more balanced lifestyle that doesn't require you to sacrifice the things you love or spend hours in the kitchen every day.

The **Low Carb, High Protein Cookbook** is more than just a collection of recipes. It's a guide to helping you understand how food affects your body, how to make smarter choices, and how to incorporate these changes into your life in a way that feels manageable and enjoyable. You'll find practical, time-saving tips for meal planning and preparation, flexible meal plans that adapt to your schedule, and delicious, easy-to-make recipes that will keep you satisfied and energized throughout the day.

One of the most important things to understand about this lifestyle is that it's not about perfection. It's about progress. You don't need to overhaul your entire diet overnight, and you certainly don't need to give up all of your favorite foods. This book is designed to help you make small, incremental changes that lead to lasting results. Whether that means starting with swapping out your usual breakfast for a protein-packed smoothie or learning how to prepare a week's worth of meals in advance so that you always have healthy options on hand, you'll find tips and strategies that meet you where you are and help you build healthier habits over time.

For many people, the biggest barrier to eating healthy is time. Between work, family, and other commitments, it can feel impossible to find the time to cook healthy meals every day. That's why this book is full of recipes that are not only nutritious but also quick and easy to make. You'll learn how to batch-cook meals that you can enjoy throughout the week, how to make the most of your leftovers, and how to prepare simple yet satisfying dishes that come together in under 30 minutes. By taking the guesswork out of meal planning and providing you with practical tools for staying organized in the kitchen, this book will help you reclaim your time while still nourishing your body with the food it needs.

In addition to practical tips and delicious recipes, this book also includes meal plans that are tailored to different goals and lifestyles. Whether you're looking to jumpstart your weight loss journey with a 28-day plan or need a more long-term 60-day solution to help you build healthier habits, you'll find flexible plans that guide you through each step of the process. These plans are designed to be adaptable, meaning you can adjust them to suit your personal preferences, family needs, or dietary restrictions. The goal is to make healthy eating feel achievable, not overwhelming.

What's more, this book takes a holistic approach to health. It's not just about what you eat, but how you approach your overall well-being. You'll find tips for staying motivated, setting realistic goals, and managing the inevitable challenges that come with making lifestyle changes. Whether you're struggling with cravings, dealing with a busy schedule, or feeling discouraged by setbacks, this book will provide you with the encouragement and support you need to stay on track.

Ultimately, this book is about empowering you to take control of your health in a way that feels sustainable and enjoyable. It's about finding balance, achieving your goals, and feeling confident in your ability to maintain your progress over the long term. You won't just learn how to follow a Low Carb, High Protein diet—you'll learn how to make it work for your life, your body, and your future.

Quick Start Guide: Making the Most of This Cookbook

Now that you have a better understanding of why the **Low Carb, High Protein** approach works and how this book can help you make meaningful changes in your life, let's dive into how to get started. This section will provide you with a **Quick Start Guide** to help you make the most of the recipes, meal plans, and tips you'll find in the following chapters.

The first step in adopting this lifestyle is to familiarize yourself with the key principles of the Low Carb, High Protein diet. As you browse through the recipes, you'll notice a common theme: meals are built around lean proteins, healthy fats, and fiber-rich vegetables, with minimal reliance on processed carbs or sugars. These recipes are designed to keep your blood sugar stable, your energy levels high, and your cravings under control.

To get started, we recommend choosing one or two meals that you can incorporate into your routine right away. Maybe that's starting your day with a protein-rich breakfast like an omelette or smoothie, or swapping out your usual sandwich at lunch for a hearty salad with grilled chicken or salmon. These small changes can have a big impact on how you feel throughout the day, and they're easy to implement without overhauling your entire routine.

Once you've started experimenting with a few recipes, take some time to explore the meal plans included in this book. Whether you're looking for a 28-day jumpstart or a more long-term 60-day plan, you'll find flexible meal plans that provide structure without feeling restrictive.

These plans are designed to be adaptable, so feel free to mix and match recipes based on your preferences, or swap in different ingredients depending on what's available to you.

Meal prep is another key strategy for success on the **Low Carb, High Protein** diet. By preparing meals in advance, you'll save time during the week and always have healthy options on hand. This book includes tips for batch cooking, storing meals, and using leftovers to make sure you're never caught without something nutritious to eat. With a little planning, you'll be able to stick to your goals even on the busiest days.

As you work your way through the recipes and meal plans, remember that flexibility is key. This book is meant to be a guide, not a strict set of rules. If you need to adjust a recipe to suit your taste preferences or make substitutions to accommodate dietary restrictions, feel free to do so. The goal is to create meals that you enjoy and that fit into your lifestyle.

Finally, don't forget to celebrate your progress. Adopting a new way of eating is a journey, and it's important to acknowledge the small wins along the way. Whether that's feeling more energetic, noticing that your clothes fit better, or simply enjoying the taste of a healthy meal, every step forward is worth celebrating.

With this Quick Start Guide, you're ready to dive into the recipes and meal plans that follow. Take your time, enjoy the process, and remember that you're building a foundation for a healthier, happier future.

CHAPTER 2

The Science Behind Low-Carb, High-Protein Eating

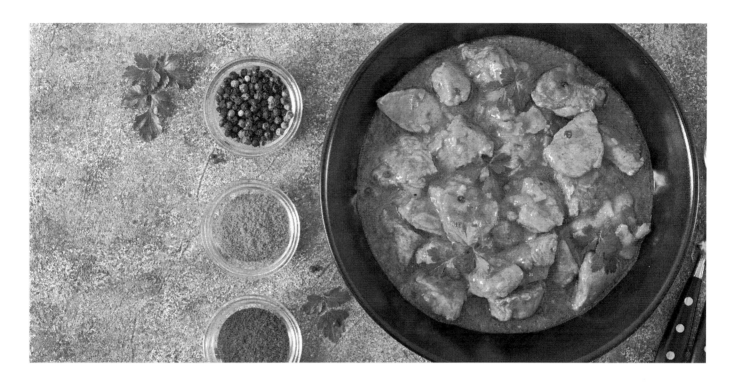

The **Low Carb, High Protein** way of eating has gained significant attention not only for its effectiveness in helping people lose weight but also for the remarkable benefits it brings in terms of muscle toning, energy levels, and overall health. While many people are initially drawn to the concept because of its promise to shed pounds, it offers far more than just a slimmer figure. The combination of lower carbohydrate intake and a boost in high-quality protein results in powerful effects that positively impact the body in a variety of ways, from enhanced metabolism to better heart health.

Understanding the science behind this way of eating will provide clarity on how it works, why it's sustainable, and why it's particularly effective for those who are busy but still want to prioritize health. This chapter will delve into the mechanisms behind **weight loss and muscle toning**, explore how this diet helps manage **hunger and cravings**, and highlight the critical **health benefits** it offers. We'll also look into how this eating plan keeps you **energized and focused** throughout the day and how it helps build **sustainable eating habits** for the long term.

Weight Loss and Muscle Toning: A Powerful Combo

For many, losing weight is the main goal when adopting a Low Carb, High Protein lifestyle. Yet, a key difference between this approach and others lies in how it allows you to lose fat while preserving or even gaining muscle. This combination is what makes the Low Carb, High Protein diet particularly appealing to people who not only want to shed weight but also tone their bodies and feel stronger in the process.

When you reduce your intake of carbohydrates, your body begins to shift from using glucose (sugar) as its primary source of energy to using stored fat. This metabolic process, known as **ketosis**, forces the body to burn fat for fuel, which accelerates weight loss. However, one of the greatest risks when losing weight is also losing muscle mass. That's where protein comes in. Protein plays a vital role in muscle repair and growth, which is particularly important when you're in a calorie deficit, which is typically required for fat loss. Protein helps ensure that the weight you're losing is primarily fat, not muscle, which is crucial for maintaining a toned appearance and keeping your metabolism high.

The synergy between lower carbs and higher protein works in a way that promotes fat loss without the accompanying muscle loss that can happen with other diets. Furthermore, protein has a thermogenic effect, meaning that your body burns more calories digesting and metabolizing protein than it does with carbs or fats. This added boost to your metabolism is yet another way this diet supports weight loss.

Muscle toning happens when you combine the right kind of exercise with the right diet. Whether you're engaging in strength training, cardio, or both, the Low Carb, High Protein approach provides your body with the nutrients it needs to recover and build muscle after workouts. The more muscle mass you maintain or build, the more calories your body burns, even at rest. This is why a higher protein intake is often associated with better long-term weight management.

Feeling Full: Managing Hunger and Cravings

One of the biggest hurdles people face when trying to lose weight is controlling hunger and cravings. Many diets that drastically reduce calorie intake leave people feeling hungry, unsatisfied, and more likely to give in to cravings. The **Low Carb, High Protein** approach offers a solution to this common issue, as it naturally helps manage appetite and keeps you feeling full longer.

Protein is well-known for its ability to suppress hunger. It takes longer to digest than carbohydrates, which means you'll feel satisfied for a more extended period after eating a high-protein meal. Additionally, protein has a significant effect on several hormones that regulate hunger and satiety. It lowers levels of the "hunger hormone" ghrelin, which tells your brain when it's time to eat. At the same time, protein increases the production of hormones like peptide YY, which signal fullness.

By incorporating more protein into your meals, you'll find that you're less prone to snack between meals or overeat at your next meal. This effect is amplified when you also reduce your intake of simple carbohydrates, which are known to cause spikes in blood sugar levels. When your blood sugar spikes and then crashes, it triggers hunger and cravings, particularly for more carbs. By cutting back on these fast-digesting carbs and replacing them with protein and healthy fats, you stabilize your blood sugar and avoid the cycle of cravings that can derail your diet.

Healthy fats, which are often included in a Low Carb, High Protein diet, also contribute to the feeling of fullness. Fats take longer to digest and don't cause the blood sugar fluctuations that carbs do. Combined with protein, fats help create balanced meals that keep your energy steady and your hunger in check, reducing the likelihood of reaching for unhealthy snacks.

Another important factor in managing hunger is **fiber**. Though the Low Carb, High Protein diet limits the intake of refined carbohydrates, it encourages the consumption of fiber-rich vegetables and certain low-carb fruits. Fiber adds bulk to your meals without adding significant calories, and it slows digestion, helping you feel full longer. Vegetables, in particular, are essential to this eating plan, as they provide necessary vitamins, minerals, and fiber without spiking blood sugar.

Health Benefits: Boosting Metabolism and Heart Health

In addition to helping with weight loss and muscle toning, the **Low Carb, High Protein** diet provides a range of health benefits that go beyond aesthetics. This eating plan supports overall metabolic health, helping your body function more efficiently while improving heart health and reducing the risk of various chronic diseases.

One of the key ways this diet boosts metabolism is through its emphasis on protein. Protein has a higher **thermic effect** than carbohydrates or fat, meaning your body burns more calories to digest and process it. This increases your overall calorie expenditure, giving your metabolism a small but meaningful boost. Additionally, maintaining or building muscle through a higher protein intake helps keep your metabolism running smoothly, as muscle tissue burns more calories than fat tissue, even at rest.

For many people, high-carbohydrate diets lead to spikes and crashes in blood sugar, which can contribute to insulin resistance over time. Insulin resistance is a precursor to type 2 diabetes and is closely linked to obesity and metabolic syndrome. By reducing the intake of refined carbohydrates and focusing on whole foods, the Low Carb, High Protein diet helps stabilize blood sugar levels and reduces the risk of developing insulin resistance. This is particularly important for people who are at risk of or are managing prediabetes or diabetes.

The diet also has positive effects on heart health. Traditional low-fat diets have long been promoted for heart health, but more recent research has shown that **low-carb diets** that include healthy fats can be even more effective in reducing heart disease risk factors. When you cut down on refined carbs and sugars, you can lower **triglyceride levels** (a type of fat in your blood) and increase **HDL cholesterol** (the "good" cholesterol), both of which are markers of improved heart health.

Healthy fats, such as those found in avocados, olive oil, nuts, seeds, and fatty fish, are essential components of the Low Carb, High Protein diet. These fats, particularly omega-3 fatty acids, help reduce inflammation in the body, which is a significant factor in the development of heart disease. By incorporating these fats into your meals while reducing unhealthy trans fats and refined carbs, you can support cardiovascular health while still enjoying rich, flavorful meals.

Staying Energized and Focused All Day

One of the biggest complaints people have about high-carb diets is the **energy rollercoaster** they experience throughout the day. After a carb-heavy meal, you might feel a burst of energy, only to crash a few hours later, feeling sluggish and in need of another quick fix. This cycle of highs and lows is exhausting, both mentally and physically, and often leads to overeating or reaching for sugary snacks for a quick energy boost.

The **Low Carb, High Protein** approach offers a solution by providing more stable, long-lasting energy throughout the day. Protein and healthy fats digest more slowly than carbohydrates, which means they offer a steady supply of energy that doesn't lead to the spikes and crashes associated with carb-heavy meals. This helps you stay energized and focused for longer periods without the need for constant snacking.

By maintaining stable blood sugar levels, this eating plan also helps improve **mental clarity** and focus. The brain relies on a steady supply of glucose for energy, but it can also use **ketones**, which are produced when the body breaks down fat. When you reduce your carb intake, your body becomes more efficient at producing and using ketones, which can help improve brain function and reduce brain fog. Many people report feeling more alert, focused, and productive after switching to a Low Carb, High Protein diet.

In addition to stabilizing blood sugar, the diet's emphasis on protein supports brain health by providing the building blocks for neurotransmitters, the chemicals that regulate mood, focus, and cognition. This combination of stable energy and improved brain function makes it easier to stay on track with your goals and maintain a positive, focused mindset throughout the day.

Another added benefit of this diet is improved **sleep quality**. Blood sugar fluctuations can interfere with sleep, causing restlessness or waking during the night. By stabilizing your blood sugar and providing your body with the nutrients it needs, the Low Carb, High Protein lifestyle helps promote more restful, uninterrupted sleep, which in turn supports better energy levels and mood during the day.

Building Sustainable Eating Habits for You and Your Family

One of the reasons why so many diets fail is that they are not sustainable in the long run. Restrictive eating plans, complicated rules, and unrealistic expectations make it difficult to stick with a diet for more than a few weeks or months. The **Low Carb, High Protein** approach, however, is designed with sustainability in mind. It encourages the adoption of healthier habits that can be maintained over time, without the need for drastic measures or constant sacrifice.

One of the key features of this eating plan is its flexibility. While the focus is on reducing carbs and increasing protein, there is plenty of room for customization based on individual preferences, dietary needs, and lifestyle factors. This makes it easier to incorporate into your daily life and more adaptable to the needs of your family. You don't need to prepare separate meals for yourself and your loved ones—the recipes in this book are designed to be family-friendly, ensuring that everyone can enjoy the same nutritious, delicious meals.

This flexibility also makes the **Low Carb, High Protein** lifestyle easier to maintain over the long term. You won't feel like you're constantly giving up the foods you love or following a rigid set of rules. Instead, you'll learn how to make smarter choices that align with your health goals without feeling deprived. Whether you're planning meals for the week, dining out, or attending social events, you'll have the knowledge and tools to make decisions that support your goals without feeling restricted.

Meal planning and preparation are central to building sustainable eating habits. By taking the time to plan your meals in advance, you'll always have healthy options on hand, making it easier to stay on track even on busy days. This book provides practical tips for meal prepping, batch cooking, and using leftovers, so you can save time in the kitchen while still enjoying nutritious, home-cooked meals.

Ultimately, the **Low Carb, High Protein** lifestyle is about creating a balanced, sustainable approach to eating that works for you and your family. It's not about perfection—it's about progress. By focusing on whole, nutrient-dense foods and making small, manageable changes over time, you'll build habits that support long-term health and well-being.

PART 2

DELICIOUS, EASY RECIPES

CHAPTER 3

Power-Up Breakfasts: Start Your Day Right

Breakfast is often called the most important meal of the day, and for good reason. It sets the tone for your energy levels, mood, and focus throughout the day. Starting your morning with a high-protein, low-carb meal ensures that you feel full and energized for hours, helping you stay on track with your health goals without feeling the need to snack or overeat.

In this chapter, we'll explore a variety of breakfast recipes that are not only delicious but also quick and easy to prepare. Whether you're in the mood for something sweet like a yogurt parfait or prefer savory options like omelettes and frittatas, these recipes are designed to kickstart your metabolism, keep you satisfied, and make mornings easier.

Each recipe is labeled with the prep time, cook time, and serving size, and comes with straightforward instructions to make your mornings less hectic. You'll also find the nutritional breakdown for each recipe, focused on the essentials: calories, fat, carbohydrates, and protein. Whether you're a busy professional, a parent, or someone looking to simplify your healthy eating routine, these breakfast recipes will power you through your day with ease and flavor.

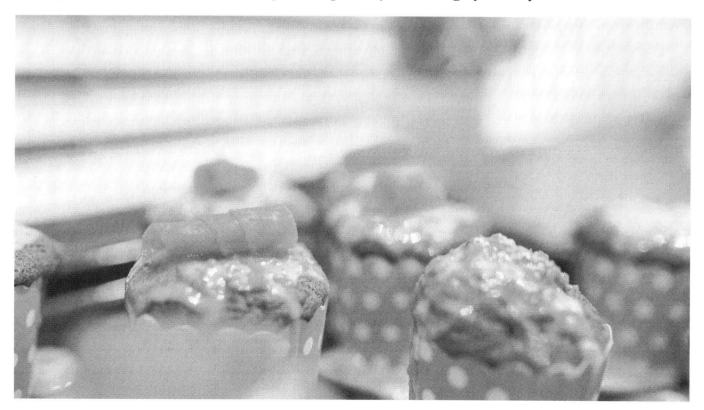

1. Greek Yogurt Parfait with Berries & Nuts

Prep: 5 minutes   **Cook: None**   **Serves: 1**

INGREDIENTS

- 1 cup plain Greek yogurt (240g)
- ½ cup mixed berries (strawberries, blueberries, raspberries)
- 2 tablespoons chopped mixed nuts (almonds, walnuts)
- 1 teaspoon chia seeds (optional)

INSTRUCTIONS

1. Spoon the Greek yogurt into a bowl or jar.
2. Layer the mixed berries on top of the yogurt.
3. Sprinkle the chopped nuts and chia seeds (if using) over the berries.
4. Serve immediately or refrigerate for later.

Nutritional Facts (Per Serving):
Calories: 250 **Fat:** 10g **Carbohydrates:** 22g **Protein:** 20g

2. Spinach & Feta Omelette

Prep: 5 minutes   **Cook: 10 minutes**   **Serves: 1**

INGREDIENTS

- 2 large eggs
- ¼ cup crumbled feta cheese (30g)
- ½ cup fresh spinach (30g)
- 1 tablespoon olive oil
- Salt and pepper to taste

INSTRUCTIONS

1. In a small bowl, whisk the eggs with a pinch of salt and pepper.
2. Heat the olive oil in a non-stick skillet over medium heat.
3. Add the spinach and cook until wilted, about 1-2 minutes.
4. Pour the whisked eggs into the skillet and cook for 2-3 minutes, until the eggs are mostly set.
5. Sprinkle the feta cheese over half of the omelette and fold the other half over. Cook for an additional minute until the cheese is slightly melted.
6. Serve hot.

Nutritional Facts (Per Serving):
Calories: 320 **Fat:** 25g **Carbohydrates:** 2g **Protein:** 18g

3. Avocado & Smoked Salmon Toast

| Prep: 5 minutes | Cook: None | Serves: 1 |

INGREDIENTS

- 1 slice of low-carb bread
- ½ avocado, mashed
- 2 oz smoked salmon (60g)
- 1 teaspoon lemon juice
- Salt and pepper to taste

INSTRUCTIONS

1. Toast the slice of low-carb bread.
2. In a small bowl, mash the avocado with lemon juice, salt, and pepper.
3. Spread the mashed avocado onto the toast.
4. Layer the smoked salmon on top of the avocado and serve.

Nutritional Facts (Per Serving):
Calories: 340 **Fat**: 25g **Carbohydrates**: 5g **Protein**: 20g

4. Cottage Cheese with Berries & Almonds

| Prep: 5 minutes | Cook: None | Serves: 1 |

INGREDIENTS

- 1 cup cottage cheese (240g)
- ½ cup mixed berries (strawberries, blueberries, raspberries)
- 1 tablespoon sliced almonds

INSTRUCTIONS

1. Spoon the cottage cheese into a bowl.
2. Top with mixed berries and sliced almonds.
3. Serve immediately.

Nutritional Facts (Per Serving):
Calories: 220 **Fat**: 9g **Carbohydrates**: 15g **Protein**: 20g

5. Scrambled Eggs with Spinach & Tomatoes

Prep: 5 minutes   **Cook: 5 minutes**   **Serves: 1**

INGREDIENTS

- 2 large eggs
- ½ cup fresh spinach (30g)
- ¼ cup cherry tomatoes, halved (40g)
- 1 tablespoon olive oil
- Salt and pepper to taste

INSTRUCTIONS

1. Heat the olive oil in a skillet over medium heat.
2. Add the spinach and cherry tomatoes, cooking until the spinach is wilted and the tomatoes are slightly softened, about 2 minutes.
3. Whisk the eggs with salt and pepper, then pour into the skillet with the vegetables.
4. Scramble the eggs for 2-3 minutes until fully cooked. Serve hot.

Nutritional Facts (Per Serving):
Calories: 270 **Fat**: 20g **Carbohydrates**: 4g **Protein**: 14g

6. Chia Seed Pudding with Almond Milk & Berries

Prep: 5 minutes   **Cook: None (overnight chill)**   **Serves: 1**

INGREDIENTS

- 3 tablespoons chia seeds
- 1 cup unsweetened almond milk
- ½ teaspoon vanilla extract
- ½ cup mixed berries (strawberries, blueberries, raspberries)
- 1 teaspoon honey or low-carb sweetener (optional)

INSTRUCTIONS

1. In a small bowl or jar, mix chia seeds, almond milk, and vanilla extract.
2. Stir well, cover, and refrigerate for at least 4 hours or overnight until the pudding thickens.
3. In the morning, top with mixed berries and honey if desired.
4. Serve chilled.

Nutritional Facts (Per Serving):
Calories: 230 **Fat**: 12g **Carbohydrates**: 20g **Protein**: 6g

7. Egg Muffins

Prep: 10 minutes	Cook: 20 minutes	Serves: 4

INGREDIENTS

- 6 large eggs
- ½ cup shredded cheese (cheddar or mozzarella)
- ½ cup chopped spinach
- ½ cup diced bell pepper
- ¼ cup chopped onions
- Salt and pepper to taste

INSTRUCTIONS

1. Preheat your oven to 375°F (190°C). Grease a muffin tin.
2. In a large bowl, whisk the eggs and season with salt and pepper.
3. Add the cheese, spinach, bell pepper, and onions to the egg mixture and stir.
4. Pour the mixture into the muffin tin, filling each cup about ¾ full.
5. Bake for 20-25 minutes or until the eggs are fully set.
6. Let cool slightly before serving.

Nutritional Facts (Per Serving):
Calories: 180 **Fat**: 12g **Carbohydrates**: 3g **Protein**: 12g

8. Oats with Almond Butter & Bananas

Prep: 5 minutes	Cook: 5 minutes	Serves: 1

INGREDIENTS

- ½ cup rolled oats
- 1 cup unsweetened almond milk
- 1 tablespoon almond butter
- ½ banana, sliced
- 1 teaspoon chia seeds (optional)

INSTRUCTIONS

1. In a small pot, bring almond milk to a boil.
2. Add rolled oats, reduce heat, and simmer for 3-5 minutes until the oats soften.
3. Remove from heat and stir in almond butter.
4. Top with sliced bananas and chia seeds if desired. Serve warm.

Nutritional Facts (Per Serving):
Calories: 320 **Fat**: 12g **Carbohydrates**: 45g **Protein**: 8g

9. Ham & Cheese Roll-Ups

Prep: 5 minutes   Cook: None   Serves: 1

INGREDIENTS

- 4 slices deli ham
- 2 slices cheddar or Swiss cheese
- 1 tablespoon mustard or mayonnaise (optional)

INSTRUCTIONS

1. Lay the slices of ham flat on a clean surface.
2. Place a slice of cheese on each piece of ham.
3. Roll each ham and cheese slice into a tight roll.
4. Serve as-is or with a side of mustard or mayonnaise for dipping.

Nutritional Facts (Per Serving):
Calories: 210 **Fat**: 14g **Carbohydrates**: 1g **Protein**: 20g

10. Protein Pancakes

Prep: 5 minutes   Cook: 10 minutes   Serves: 2

INGREDIENTS

- 1 scoop vanilla protein powder
- 1 large egg
- ¼ cup almond flour
- ¼ cup unsweetened almond milk
- 1 teaspoon baking powder
- ½ teaspoon vanilla extract
- Butter or coconut oil for cooking

INSTRUCTIONS

1. In a bowl, whisk together protein powder, egg, almond flour, almond milk, baking powder, and vanilla extract.
2. Heat a skillet over medium heat and melt a small amount of butter or coconut oil.
3. Pour batter onto the skillet, making small pancakes.
4. Cook for 2-3 minutes on each side until golden brown.
5. Serve with sugar-free syrup or fresh berries.

Nutritional Facts (Per Serving):
Calories: 270 **Fat**: 15g **Carbohydrates**: 5g **Protein**: 25g

11. Burritos

Prep: 10 minutes   Cook: 5 minutes   Serves: 2

INGREDIENTS

- 4 large eggs
- 2 low-carb tortillas
- ¼ cup shredded cheese
- 2 tablespoons salsa
- 1 tablespoon butter

INSTRUCTIONS

1. In a bowl, whisk the eggs.
2. Heat butter in a skillet over medium heat. Scramble the eggs until cooked through.
3. Warm the tortillas in a separate pan or microwave.
4. Divide scrambled eggs, shredded cheese, and salsa between the two tortillas.
5. Roll the tortillas into burritos and serve hot.

Nutritional Facts (Per Serving):
Calories: 320 **Fat**: 18g **Carbohydrates**: 10g **Protein**: 20g

12. Sausage & Egg Skillet

Prep: 5 minutes   Cook: 15 minutes   Serves: 1

INGREDIENTS

- 2 sausage links (chicken or turkey)
- 2 large eggs
- ¼ cup diced bell peppers
- ¼ cup diced onions
- 1 tablespoon olive oil

INSTRUCTIONS

1. Heat olive oil in a skillet over medium heat. Add sausage links and cook for 5-7 minutes, turning occasionally.
2. Add the bell peppers and onions to the skillet and cook for 2-3 minutes.
3. Crack the eggs into the skillet and cook until the whites are set but the yolks are still runny.
4. Serve immediately.

Nutritional Facts (Per Serving):
Calories: 400 **Fat**: 30g **Carbohydrates**: 4g **Protein**: 25g

13. Turkey Bacon & Egg Cups

Prep: 10 minutes   **Cook: 15 minutes**   **Serves: 4**

INGREDIENTS

- 8 slices turkey bacon
- 8 large eggs
- Salt and pepper to taste
- ¼ cup shredded cheese (optional)

INSTRUCTIONS

1. Preheat the oven to 350°F (175°C). Grease a muffin tin.
2. Line each muffin cup with a slice of turkey bacon.
3. Crack an egg into each bacon-lined cup. Sprinkle with salt, pepper, and cheese (if using).
4. Bake for 12-15 minutes, or until the egg whites are set.
5. Serve warm.

Nutritional Facts (Per Serving):
Calories: 120 **Fat:** 8g **Carbohydrates:** 1g **Protein:** 10g

14. Low-Carb Pizza

Prep: 10 minutes   **Cook: 15 minutes**   **Serves: 2**

INGREDIENTS

- ½ cup almond flour
- 1 egg
- ½ cup shredded mozzarella
- 2 tablespoons pizza sauce (sugar-free)
- ¼ cup toppings of choice (pepperoni, mushrooms, etc.)

INSTRUCTIONS

1. Preheat your oven to 375°F (190°C). Line a baking sheet with parchment paper.
2. In a bowl, mix almond flour, egg, and mozzarella to form the dough.
3. Press the dough into a circle on the prepared baking sheet.
4. Bake for 10 minutes until the edges are slightly golden.
5. Remove from the oven, add pizza sauce and toppings, and bake for another 5 minutes.
6. Slice and serve hot.

Nutritional Facts (Per Serving):
Calories: 320 **Fat:** 22g **Carbohydrates:** 5g **Protein:** 20g

15. Salmon & Asparagus Frittata

Prep: 10 minutes   **Cook: 15 minutes**   **Serves: 2**

INGREDIENTS

- 4 large eggs
- ½ cup cooked salmon, flaked
- ½ cup cooked asparagus, chopped
- 2 tablespoons olive oil
- Salt and pepper to taste

INSTRUCTIONS

1. Preheat the oven to 375°F (190°C).
2. Heat olive oil in a skillet over medium heat.
3. In a bowl, whisk the eggs with salt and pepper.
4. Add the salmon and asparagus to the skillet, then pour in the whisked eggs.
5. Cook for 5 minutes on the stove, then transfer the skillet to the oven.
6. Bake for 10 minutes or until the eggs are fully set.
7. Serve warm.

Nutritional Facts (Per Serving):
Calories: 280 **Fat**: 18g **Carbohydrates**: 2g **Protein**: 25g

CHAPTER 4

Healthy and Fast Lunches

Lunch is a critical meal of the day that often needs to strike a balance between being quick to prepare and providing the energy you need to power through the afternoon. The recipes in this chapter are designed to be both nutritious and satisfying, keeping you full and energized without requiring too much time in the kitchen. Whether you're packing a lunch for work, looking for a healthy meal to whip up at home, or preparing something easy for the family, these options offer flexibility and flavor.

From hearty salads to wraps, stir-fries, and nutrient-packed bowls, you'll find a range of recipes that cater to your low-carb, high-protein lifestyle. Let's dive into these 15 delicious lunch recipes!

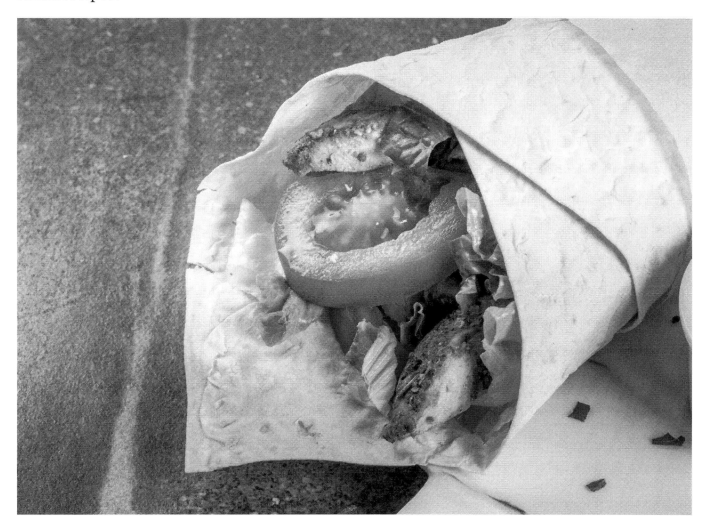

16. Grilled Chicken Caesar Salad

Prep: 10 minutes	Cook: 10 minutes	Serves: 2

INGREDIENTS

- 2 boneless, skinless chicken breasts
- 4 cups chopped romaine lettuce
- ¼ cup grated Parmesan cheese
- 2 tablespoons Caesar dressing (low-carb)
- 1 tablespoon olive oil
- Salt and pepper to taste
- Optional: ½ cup croutons (for non-low-carb option)

INSTRUCTIONS

1. Heat a grill pan or outdoor grill to medium-high heat. Brush the chicken breasts with olive oil, and season with salt and pepper.
2. Grill the chicken for 5-7 minutes per side, or until fully cooked.
3. In a large bowl, combine chopped romaine lettuce, Parmesan cheese, and Caesar dressing.
4. Slice the grilled chicken and place it on top of the salad. Serve immediately.

Nutritional Facts (Per Serving):
Calories: 320 **Fat:** 20g **Carbohydrates:** 4g **Protein:** 30g

17. Turkey Avocado Wrap

Prep: 5 minutes	Cook: None	Serves: 1

INGREDIENTS

- 1 low-carb tortilla
- 3 slices deli turkey breast
- ¼ avocado, sliced
- 1 tablespoon mayonnaise
- 1 slice Swiss cheese
- Lettuce leaves

INSTRUCTIONS

1. Spread mayonnaise onto the low-carb tortilla.
2. Layer the turkey, avocado slices, Swiss cheese, and lettuce leaves on the tortilla.
3. Roll the tortilla tightly into a wrap, slice in half, and serve.

Nutritional Facts (Per Serving):
Calories: 350 **Fat:** 25g **Carbohydrates:** 7g **Protein:** 22g

18. Baked Salmon with Dill & Lemon

Prep: 5 minutes   **Cook: 15 minutes**   **Serves: 2**

INGREDIENTS

- 2 salmon fillets (6 oz each)
- 2 tablespoons fresh dill, chopped
- 1 lemon, sliced
- 1 tablespoon olive oil
- Salt and pepper to taste

INSTRUCTIONS

1. Preheat the oven to 400°F (200°C). Line a baking sheet with parchment paper.
2. Place the salmon fillets on the sheet, drizzle with olive oil, and sprinkle with dill, salt, and pepper.
3. Top each fillet with a couple of lemon slices.
4. Bake for 12-15 minutes or until the salmon is cooked through and flakes easily with a fork.
5. Serve with extra lemon slices if desired.

Nutritional Facts (Per Serving):
Calories: 310 **Fat**: 20g **Carbohydrates**: 2g **Protein**: 28g

19. Eggplant Lasagna

Prep: 15 minutes   **Cook: 45 minutes**   **Serves: 4**

INGREDIENTS

- 2 large eggplants, sliced lengthwise
- 1 lb ground beef or turkey
- 2 cups marinara sauce (sugar-free)
- 2 cups ricotta cheese
- 1 cup shredded mozzarella
- 1 egg
- 1 tablespoon olive oil
- Salt and pepper to taste

INSTRUCTIONS

1. Preheat the oven to 375°F (190°C). Grease a baking dish.
2. Heat olive oil in a pan and cook the ground beef or turkey until browned. Add marinara sauce and simmer for 5 minutes.
3. In a bowl, mix ricotta cheese, egg, salt, and pepper.
4. Layer the sliced eggplant in the baking dish, followed by the meat sauce, ricotta mixture, and a sprinkle of mozzarella cheese.
5. Repeat the layers until all ingredients are used. Finish with a top layer of mozzarella.
6. Cover with foil and bake for 30 minutes. Remove the foil and bake for an additional 15 minutes until the cheese is golden.
7. Let it cool slightly before serving.

Nutritional Facts (Per Serving):
Calories: 380 **Fat**: 25g **Carbohydrates**: 12g **Protein**: 30g

20. Shrimp & Avocado Salad

Prep: 10 minutes	Cook: 5 minutes	Serves: 2

INGREDIENTS

- 1 lb shrimp, peeled and deveined
- 1 avocado, diced
- 4 cups mixed greens
- 1 tablespoon olive oil
- Juice of 1 lime
- Salt and pepper to taste

INSTRUCTIONS

1. Heat olive oil in a skillet over medium heat. Add shrimp and cook for 3-5 minutes until pink and cooked through.
2. In a large bowl, toss mixed greens, avocado, and cooked shrimp.
3. Drizzle with lime juice, season with salt and pepper, and serve.

Nutritional Facts (Per Serving):
Calories: 290 **Fat**: 18g **Carbohydrates**: 8g **Protein**: 25g

21. Grilled Chicken & Pesto Wrap

Prep: 10 minutes	Cook: 10 minutes	Serves: 2

INGREDIENTS

- 2 boneless, skinless chicken breasts
- 2 low-carb tortillas
- 2 tablespoons pesto sauce
- ½ cup shredded mozzarella cheese
- 1 cup spinach leaves
- 1 tablespoon olive oil

INSTRUCTIONS

1. Heat olive oil in a grill pan and cook chicken breasts for 5-7 minutes per side until fully cooked.
2. Slice the chicken and divide it between the tortillas.
3. Spread pesto sauce on each tortilla, add mozzarella and spinach, and roll into wraps.
4. Serve warm.

Nutritional Facts (Per Serving):
Calories: 400 **Fat**: 24g **Carbohydrates**: 10g **Protein**: 30g

22. Chicken & Vegetable Skewers

Prep: 10 minutes   Cook: 15 minutes   Serves: 2

INGREDIENTS

- 2 boneless, skinless chicken breasts, cut into cubes
- 1 bell pepper, cut into chunks
- 1 zucchini, sliced into rounds
- 1 red onion, cut into wedges
- 2 tablespoons olive oil
- Salt and pepper to taste

INSTRUCTIONS

1. Preheat a grill to medium-high heat. Thread chicken, bell pepper, zucchini, and onion onto skewers.
2. Brush with olive oil and season with salt and pepper.
3. Grill the skewers for 10-15 minutes, turning occasionally, until the chicken is cooked through.
4. Serve immediately.

Nutritional Facts (Per Serving):
Calories: 320 **Fat**: 14g **Carbohydrates**: 8g **Protein**: 35g

23. Kale & Quinoa Salad

Prep: 10 minutes   Cook: 15 minutes   Serves: 2

INGREDIENTS

- 1 cup cooked quinoa
- 2 cups chopped kale
- ¼ cup crumbled feta cheese
- 2 tablespoons olive oil
- Juice of 1 lemon
- Salt and pepper to taste

INSTRUCTIONS

1. In a large bowl, toss cooked quinoa, chopped kale, and feta cheese.
2. Drizzle with olive oil and lemon juice, and season with salt and pepper.
3. Serve immediately.

Nutritional Facts (Per Serving):
Calories: 250 **Fat**: 12g **Carbohydrates**: 22g **Protein**: 10g

24. Spaghetti Squash with Meatballs

Prep: 10 minutes	Cook: 40 minutes	Serves: 2

INGREDIENTS

- 1 small spaghetti squash
- ½ lb ground beef or turkey
- 1 egg
- ¼ cup grated Parmesan cheese
- 1 cup marinara sauce (sugar-free)
- 1 tablespoon olive oil
- Salt and pepper to taste

INSTRUCTIONS

1. Preheat the oven to 400°F (200°C). Slice the spaghetti squash in half, scoop out the seeds, and place it face down on a baking sheet. Roast for 30-40 minutes or until tender.
2. In a bowl, mix ground beef, egg, Parmesan, salt, and pepper. Form into meatballs.
3. Heat olive oil in a pan and cook the meatballs for 8-10 minutes, until browned and cooked through.
4. Heat the marinara sauce and add the cooked meatballs.
5. Once the squash is cooked, scrape out the strands with a fork and serve topped with meatballs and sauce.

Nutritional Facts (Per Serving):
Calories: 350 **Fat:** 18g **Carbohydrates:** 18g **Protein:** 28g

25. Tuna Avocado Sandwich

Prep: 5 minutes	Cook: None	Serves: 1

INGREDIENTS

- 1 can tuna in water, drained
- ½ avocado, mashed
- 1 tablespoon mayonnaise
- 2 slices low-carb bread
- Salt and pepper to taste

INSTRUCTIONS

1. In a bowl, mix tuna, mashed avocado, and mayonnaise. Season with salt and pepper.
2. Spread the mixture between two slices of low-carb bread.
3. Serve immediately.

Nutritional Facts (Per Serving):
Calories: 320 **Fat:** 20g **Carbohydrates:** 5g **Protein:** 25g

26. Spicy Shrimp Lettuce Wraps

Prep: 10 minutes   Cook: 5 minutes   Serves: 2

INGREDIENTS

- 1 lb shrimp, peeled and deveined
- 1 tablespoon hot sauce
- 8 large lettuce leaves (butter or romaine)
- 1 tablespoon olive oil
- Salt and pepper to taste

INSTRUCTIONS

1. Heat olive oil in a skillet over medium heat. Add shrimp and hot sauce, cooking for 3-5 minutes until shrimp are fully cooked.
2. Spoon the shrimp into lettuce leaves, season with salt and pepper, and serve.

Nutritional Facts (Per Serving):
Calories: 220 **Fat**: 10g **Carbohydrates**: 4g **Protein**: 28g

27. Zucchini Noodles with Pesto & Chicken

Prep: 10 minutes   Cook: 10 minutes   Serves: 2

INGREDIENTS

- 2 boneless, skinless chicken breasts, sliced
- 2 zucchinis, spiralized into noodles
- ¼ cup pesto sauce
- 1 tablespoon olive oil
- Salt and pepper to taste

INSTRUCTIONS

1. Heat olive oil in a skillet over medium heat. Cook the chicken slices for 6-8 minutes until fully cooked.
2. Add the zucchini noodles to the skillet and toss with the chicken for 2-3 minutes.
3. Stir in the pesto sauce and season with salt and pepper. Serve immediately.

Nutritional Facts (Per Serving):
Calories: 350 **Fat**: 24g **Carbohydrates**: 7g **Protein**: 28g

28. Asian Chicken Salad

| Prep: 10 minutes | Cook: 10 minutes | Serves: 2 |

INGREDIENTS

- 2 boneless, skinless chicken breasts
- 4 cups shredded cabbage
- 1 carrot, grated
- 2 tablespoons soy sauce (low-sodium)
- 1 tablespoon sesame oil
- 1 tablespoon rice vinegar
- 1 tablespoon sesame seeds

INSTRUCTIONS

1. Heat a skillet over medium heat and cook the chicken breasts for 6-8 minutes per side until fully cooked. Slice thinly.
2. In a large bowl, toss shredded cabbage, carrot, soy sauce, sesame oil, and rice vinegar.
3. Top with sliced chicken and sprinkle with sesame seeds. Serve immediately.

Nutritional Facts (Per Serving):
Calories: 290 **Fat**: 14g **Carbohydrates**: 8g **Protein**: 28g

29. Eggplant & Hummus Wrap

| Prep: 10 minutes | Cook: 10 minutes | Serves: 1 |

INGREDIENTS

- 2 slices grilled eggplant
- 2 tablespoons hummus
- 1 low-carb tortilla
- 1 tablespoon olive oil
- Salt and pepper to taste

INSTRUCTIONS

1. Grill the eggplant slices in a pan with olive oil for 5 minutes on each side.
2. Spread hummus on the low-carb tortilla, then add the grilled eggplant.
3. Roll the tortilla into a wrap, slice in half, and serve.

Nutritional Facts (Per Serving):
Calories: 230 **Fat**: 12g **Carbohydrates**: 15g **Protein**: 8g

30. Beef & Vegetable Stir-Fry

Prep: 10 minutes   **Cook: 10 minutes**   **Serves: 2**

INGREDIENTS

- ½ lb beef sirloin, sliced thinly
- 1 bell pepper, sliced
- 1 zucchini, sliced
- 1 tablespoon soy sauce (low-sodium)
- 1 tablespoon olive oil
- Salt and pepper to taste

INSTRUCTIONS

1. Heat olive oil in a wok or large pan over high heat. Add beef slices and cook for 3-4 minutes until browned.
2. Add bell pepper and zucchini, stir-frying for another 3-4 minutes until tender.
3. Stir in soy sauce, season with salt and pepper, and serve hot.

Nutritional Facts (Per Serving):
Calories: 320 **Fat**: 20g **Carbohydrates**: 8g **Protein**: 28g

CHAPTER 5
Family-Friendly Dinners

Dinners are the perfect opportunity to bring the family together around a meal that is not only delicious but also healthy and satisfying. In this chapter, you'll find a selection of family-friendly recipes that cater to a wide variety of tastes, while keeping them low-carb and high-protein. Whether you're cooking for picky eaters or serving a crowd, these dinners are quick to prepare and packed with flavor. From juicy steaks to zoodles and casseroles, these meals ensure everyone leaves the table happy.

Each recipe is crafted to be nutritious, filling, and perfect for dinner, making weeknights easier and more enjoyable. Let's get into these 20 mouthwatering dinners!

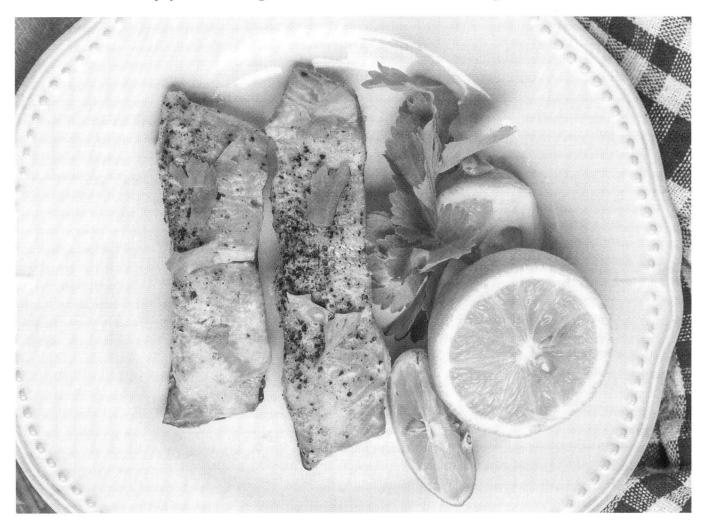

31. Grilled Steak with Chimichurri Sauce

Prep: 10 minutes | **Cook: 10 minutes** | **Serves: 2**

INGREDIENTS

- 2 ribeye steaks
- ½ cup fresh parsley, finely chopped
- 2 garlic cloves, minced
- ¼ cup olive oil
- 2 tablespoons red wine vinegar
- 1 teaspoon red pepper flakes
- Salt and pepper to taste

INSTRUCTIONS

1. Preheat a grill to medium-high heat. Season steaks with salt and pepper.
2. Grill the steaks for 4-5 minutes on each side, or until they reach your desired doneness.
3. In a small bowl, mix parsley, garlic, olive oil, vinegar, red pepper flakes, salt, and pepper to make the chimichurri sauce.
4. Let the steaks rest for 5 minutes, then drizzle with chimichurri sauce. Serve.

Nutritional Facts (Per Serving):
Calories: 450 **Fat**: 32g **Carbohydrates**: 3g **Protein**: 35g

32. Baked Lemon Herb Salmon

Prep: 5 minutes | **Cook: 15 minutes** | **Serves: 2**

INGREDIENTS

- 2 salmon fillets (6 oz each)
- 1 tablespoon olive oil
- Juice of 1 lemon
- 1 tablespoon fresh parsley, chopped
- 1 garlic clove, minced
- Salt and pepper to taste

INSTRUCTIONS

1. Preheat the oven to 400°F (200°C).
2. Place the salmon fillets on a lined baking sheet. Drizzle with olive oil and lemon juice, and sprinkle with parsley, garlic, salt, and pepper.
3. Bake for 12-15 minutes, or until the salmon flakes easily with a fork. Serve hot.

Nutritional Facts (Per Serving):
Calories: 350 **Fat**: 25g **Carbohydrates**: 2g **Protein**: 28g

33. Balsamic Glazed Chicken

Prep: 10 minutes   Cook: 20 minutes   Serves: 4

INGREDIENTS

- 4 boneless, skinless chicken breasts
- ¼ cup balsamic vinegar
- 1 tablespoon honey or sugar-free sweetener
- 1 tablespoon olive oil
- 1 garlic clove, minced
- Salt and pepper to taste

INSTRUCTIONS

1. In a small bowl, mix balsamic vinegar, honey, and garlic.
2. Heat olive oil in a skillet over medium heat. Season chicken breasts with salt and pepper, then add to the skillet. Cook for 5-6 minutes per side.
3. Pour the balsamic glaze over the chicken and cook for an additional 5 minutes, until the glaze thickens and the chicken is fully cooked.
4. Serve with extra glaze drizzled on top.

Nutritional Facts (Per Serving):
Calories: 280 **Fat**: 10g **Carbohydrates**: 6g **Protein**: 35g

34. Lemon Garlic Shrimp Pasta

Prep: 10 minutes   Cook: 10 minutes   Serves: 2

INGREDIENTS

- 8 oz shrimp, peeled and deveined
- 2 zucchinis, spiralized into noodles
- 2 tablespoons olive oil
- 2 garlic cloves, minced
- Juice of 1 lemon
- 1 tablespoon fresh parsley, chopped
- Salt and pepper to taste

INSTRUCTIONS

1. Heat olive oil in a skillet over medium heat. Add garlic and cook for 1-2 minutes.
2. Add shrimp to the skillet and cook until pink, about 3-5 minutes.
3. Stir in lemon juice and parsley.
4. Add zucchini noodles to the skillet and toss with the shrimp and sauce. Cook for another 2-3 minutes, until the zoodles are tender. Serve hot.

Nutritional Facts (Per Serving):
Calories: 230 **Fat**: 14g **Carbohydrates**: 6g **Protein**: 20g

35. Pesto Zoodles with Chicken

Prep: 10 minutes   Cook: 10 minutes   Serves: 2

INGREDIENTS

- 2 boneless, skinless chicken breasts, sliced
- 2 zucchinis, spiralized into noodles
- ¼ cup pesto sauce
- 1 tablespoon olive oil
- Salt and pepper to taste

INSTRUCTIONS

1. Heat olive oil in a skillet over medium heat. Cook the chicken slices for 6-8 minutes, until fully cooked.
2. Add the zucchini noodles to the skillet and toss with the chicken for 2-3 minutes.
3. Stir in the pesto sauce and season with salt and pepper. Serve immediately.

Nutritional Facts (Per Serving):
Calories: 350 **Fat**: 24g **Carbohydrates**: 7g **Protein**: 28g

36. Garlic Butter Shrimp with Asparagus

Prep: 10 minutes   Cook: 10 minutes   Serves: 2

INGREDIENTS

- 8 oz shrimp, peeled and deveined
- 1 bunch asparagus, trimmed
- 2 tablespoons butter
- 2 garlic cloves, minced
- Salt and pepper to taste

INSTRUCTIONS

1. Melt butter in a skillet over medium heat. Add garlic and cook for 1-2 minutes.
2. Add shrimp and asparagus to the skillet. Cook for 3-5 minutes, until shrimp are pink and the asparagus is tender.
3. Season with salt and pepper. Serve immediately.

Nutritional Facts (Per Serving):
Calories: 250 **Fat**: 18g **Carbohydrates**: 5g **Protein**: 20g

37. Lamb Chops with Mint Yogurt Sauce

| Prep: 10 minutes | Cook: 10 minutes | Serves: 2 |

INGREDIENTS

- 4 lamb chops
- 1 tablespoon olive oil
- Salt and pepper to taste
- ½ cup Greek yogurt
- 2 tablespoons fresh mint, chopped
- 1 tablespoon lemon juice

INSTRUCTIONS

1. Heat olive oil in a skillet over medium-high heat. Season lamb chops with salt and pepper.
2. Sear the lamb chops for 4-5 minutes per side, until browned and cooked to your liking.
3. In a small bowl, mix yogurt, mint, and lemon juice to make the mint yogurt sauce.
4. Serve the lamb chops with the yogurt sauce on the side.

Nutritional Facts (Per Serving):
Calories: 370 **Fat:** 25g **Carbohydrates:** 3g **Protein:** 30g

38. Garlic Parmesan Crusted Chicken

| Prep: 10 minutes | Cook: 20 minutes | Serves: 2 |

INGREDIENTS

- 2 boneless, skinless chicken breasts
- ¼ cup grated Parmesan cheese
- ¼ cup almond flour
- 1 egg, beaten
- 1 tablespoon olive oil
- 1 garlic clove, minced
- Salt and pepper to taste

INSTRUCTIONS

1. In a bowl, mix Parmesan, almond flour, garlic, salt, and pepper.
2. Dip each chicken breast in the beaten egg, then coat with the Parmesan mixture.
3. Heat olive oil in a skillet over medium heat and cook the chicken for 5-6 minutes per side, until golden and cooked through.
4. Serve immediately.

Nutritional Facts (Per Serving):
Calories: 350 **Fat:** 22g **Carbohydrates:** 5g **Protein:** 30g

39. Creamy Tuscan Garlic Chicken

Prep: 10 minutes   Cook: 20 minutes   Serves: 2

INGREDIENTS

- 2 boneless, skinless chicken breasts
- 1 tablespoon olive oil
- 1 garlic clove, minced
- ½ cup heavy cream
- ½ cup sun-dried tomatoes
- 1 cup spinach
- Salt and pepper to taste

INSTRUCTIONS

1. Heat olive oil in a skillet over medium heat. Add chicken breasts and cook for 5-6 minutes per side.
2. Remove chicken and set aside. In the same skillet, sauté garlic for 1-2 minutes.
3. Stir in heavy cream, sun-dried tomatoes, and spinach. Cook for 2-3 minutes until the spinach wilts.
4. Return the chicken to the skillet and simmer in the sauce for an additional 5 minutes. Serve hot.

Nutritional Facts (Per Serving):
Calories: 420 **Fat**: 28g **Carbohydrates**: 7g **Protein**: 35g

40. Cajun Chicken & Cauliflower Rice

Prep: 10 minutes   Cook: 15 minutes   Serves: 2

INGREDIENTS

- 2 boneless, skinless chicken breasts, sliced
- 2 cups cauliflower rice
- 1 tablespoon Cajun seasoning
- 1 tablespoon olive oil
- Salt and pepper to taste

INSTRUCTIONS

1. Heat olive oil in a skillet over medium heat. Add the chicken slices and season with Cajun seasoning. Cook for 6-8 minutes, until fully cooked.
2. Add cauliflower rice to the skillet and stir-fry for 3-4 minutes.
3. Season with salt and pepper. Serve immediately.

Nutritional Facts (Per Serving):
Calories: 300 **Fat**: 18g **Carbohydrates**: 6g **Protein**: 28g

41. Chicken Sausage & Peppers

Prep: 10 minutes   **Cook: 15 minutes**   **Serves: 2**

INGREDIENTS

- 4 chicken sausages, sliced
- 1 bell pepper, sliced
- 1 onion, sliced
- 1 tablespoon olive oil
- 1 teaspoon Italian seasoning
- Salt and pepper to taste

INSTRUCTIONS

1. Heat olive oil in a skillet over medium heat. Add sausages, bell pepper, and onion.
2. Cook for 10-12 minutes until the sausages are browned and the vegetables are tender.
3. Season with Italian seasoning, salt, and pepper. Serve hot.

Nutritional Facts (Per Serving):
Calories: 320 **Fat**: 20g **Carbohydrates**: 6g **Protein**: 25g

42. Teriyaki Salmon

Prep: 5 minutes   **Cook: 10 minutes**   **Serves: 2**

INGREDIENTS

- 2 salmon fillets (6 oz each)
- ¼ cup soy sauce (low-sodium)
- 1 tablespoon honey or sugar-free sweetener
- 1 tablespoon rice vinegar
- 1 teaspoon sesame oil
- 1 teaspoon grated ginger

INSTRUCTIONS

1. In a small bowl, whisk together soy sauce, honey, rice vinegar, sesame oil, and ginger.
2. Heat a skillet over medium heat and sear the salmon for 3-4 minutes per side.
3. Pour the teriyaki sauce over the salmon and cook for another 2 minutes until the sauce thickens.
4. Serve immediately with extra sauce drizzled on top.

Nutritional Facts (Per Serving):
Calories: 340 **Fat**: 22g **Carbohydrates**: 7g **Protein**: 25g

43. Coconut Curry Chicken

Prep: 10 minutes   Cook: 20 minutes   Serves: 2

INGREDIENTS

- 2 boneless, skinless chicken breasts, sliced
- 1 tablespoon curry powder
- 1 can (13.5 oz) coconut milk
- 1 tablespoon olive oil
- 1 garlic clove, minced
- 1 cup chopped spinach
- Salt and pepper to taste

INSTRUCTIONS

1. Heat olive oil in a skillet over medium heat. Add garlic and cook for 1-2 minutes.
2. Add chicken and curry powder, cooking for 5-6 minutes.
3. Stir in coconut milk and spinach. Simmer for 10 minutes until the sauce thickens and the chicken is cooked through.
4. Serve hot.

Nutritional Facts (Per Serving):
Calories: 400 **Fat**: 30g **Carbohydrates**: 5g **Protein**: 28g

44. Beef Fajita Bowls

Prep: 10 minutes   Cook: 10 minutes   Serves: 2

INGREDIENTS

- ½ lb beef sirloin, sliced thinly
- 1 bell pepper, sliced
- 1 onion, sliced
- 1 tablespoon fajita seasoning
- 1 tablespoon olive oil
- 2 cups cauliflower rice
- Salt and pepper to taste

INSTRUCTIONS

1. Heat olive oil in a skillet over high heat. Add beef, bell pepper, and onion. Cook for 6-8 minutes, until the beef is browned and the vegetables are tender.
2. Stir in fajita seasoning and cook for another minute.
3. Serve the beef mixture over cauliflower rice.

Nutritional Facts (Per Serving):
Calories: 350 **Fat**: 22g **Carbohydrates**: 7g **Protein**: 28g

45. Garlic Butter Steak Bites

Prep: 5 minutes   **Cook: 5 minutes**   **Serves: 2**

INGREDIENTS

- ½ lb steak, cubed
- 2 tablespoons butter
- 2 garlic cloves, minced
- Salt and pepper to taste

INSTRUCTIONS

1. Melt butter in a skillet over medium heat. Add garlic and cook for 1-2 minutes.
2. Add steak cubes and sear for 3-4 minutes, turning to cook on all sides.
3. Season with salt and pepper, and serve immediately.

Nutritional Facts (Per Serving):
Calories: 320 **Fat**: 25g **Carbohydrates**: 3g **Protein**: 25g

46. Thai Coconut Chicken Curry

Prep: 10 minutes   **Cook: 20 minutes**   **Serves: 2**

INGREDIENTS

- 2 boneless, skinless chicken breasts, sliced
- 1 tablespoon red curry paste
- 1 can (13.5 oz) coconut milk
- 1 tablespoon olive oil
- 1 garlic clove, minced
- 1 cup chopped bell pepper
- Salt and pepper to taste

INSTRUCTIONS

1. Heat olive oil in a skillet over medium heat. Add garlic and cook for 1-2 minutes.
2. Add chicken and red curry paste, cooking for 5-6 minutes.
3. Stir in coconut milk and bell pepper. Simmer for 10 minutes until the sauce thickens and the chicken is cooked through.
4. Serve hot.

Nutritional Facts (Per Serving):
Calories: 420 **Fat**: 30g **Carbohydrates**: 6g **Protein**: 28g

47. Lemon Dill Baked Cod

| Prep: 5 minutes | Cook: 15 minutes | Serves: 2 |

INGREDIENTS

- 2 cod fillets
- 1 tablespoon olive oil
- Juice of 1 lemon
- 1 tablespoon fresh dill, chopped
- Salt and pepper to taste

INSTRUCTIONS

1. Preheat the oven to 400°F (200°C). Line a baking sheet with parchment paper.
2. Place the cod fillets on the baking sheet. Drizzle with olive oil and lemon juice, and sprinkle with dill, salt, and pepper.
3. Bake for 12-15 minutes, or until the fish flakes easily with a fork. Serve hot.

Nutritional Facts (Per Serving):
Calories: 250 **Fat**: 15g **Carbohydrates**: 2g **Protein**: 25g

48. Keto Chicken Alfredo Casserole

| Prep: 10 minutes | Cook: 20 minutes | Serves: 4 |

INGREDIENTS

- 2 cups cooked chicken, shredded
- 1 cup heavy cream
- ½ cup grated Parmesan cheese
- 1 cup spinach
- 1 tablespoon olive oil
- Salt and pepper to taste

INSTRUCTIONS

1. Preheat the oven to 375°F (190°C). Grease a baking dish.
2. In a skillet, heat olive oil and sauté spinach until wilted.
3. In a bowl, mix chicken, heavy cream, Parmesan, and cooked spinach. Season with salt and pepper.
4. Pour the mixture into the baking dish and bake for 15-20 minutes, until golden and bubbly. Serve hot.

Nutritional Facts (Per Serving):
Calories: 320 **Fat**: 25g **Carbohydrates**: 3g **Protein**: 20g

49. Pesto Shrimp Zoodles

Prep: 10 minutes	Cook: 10 minutes	Serves: 2

INGREDIENTS

- 8 oz shrimp, peeled and deveined
- 2 zucchinis, spiralized into noodles
- ¼ cup pesto sauce
- 1 tablespoon olive oil
- Salt and pepper to taste

INSTRUCTIONS

1. Heat olive oil in a skillet over medium heat. Cook the shrimp for 3-5 minutes until pink.
2. Add the zucchini noodles to the skillet and toss with shrimp for 2-3 minutes.
3. Stir in the pesto sauce and season with salt and pepper. Serve immediately.

Nutritional Facts (Per Serving):
Calories: 300 **Fat:** 20g **Carbohydrates:** 7g **Protein:** 24g

50. Beef Stir-Fry

Prep: 10 minutes	Cook: 10 minutes	Serves: 2

INGREDIENTS

- ½ lb beef sirloin, sliced thinly
- 1 bell pepper, sliced
- 1 zucchini, sliced
- 1 tablespoon soy sauce (low-sodium)
- 1 tablespoon olive oil
- Salt and pepper to taste

INSTRUCTIONS

1. Heat olive oil in a wok or large pan over high heat. Add beef slices and cook for 3-4 minutes until browned.
2. Add bell pepper and zucchini, stir-frying for another 3-4 minutes until tender.
3. Stir in soy sauce, season with salt and pepper, and serve hot.

Nutritional Facts (Per Serving):
Calories: 320 **Fat:** 20g **Carbohydrates:** 8g **Protein:** 28g

CHAPTER 6
Guilt-Free Treats: Desserts and Snacks

Who says you have to give up your favorite treats to stay on track with a low-carb, high-protein lifestyle? In this chapter, we'll explore delicious, guilt-free desserts and snacks that satisfy your sweet tooth without derailing your health goals. Whether you're craving a quick snack, a protein-packed bite, or a decadent dessert, these recipes are designed to provide all the indulgence without the guilt.

These treats are packed with healthy fats, protein, and low in refined sugars, making them the perfect addition to your diet. From protein balls to brownies and cookies, let's dive into these 25 delicious recipes that prove healthy eating can be both satisfying and delicious!

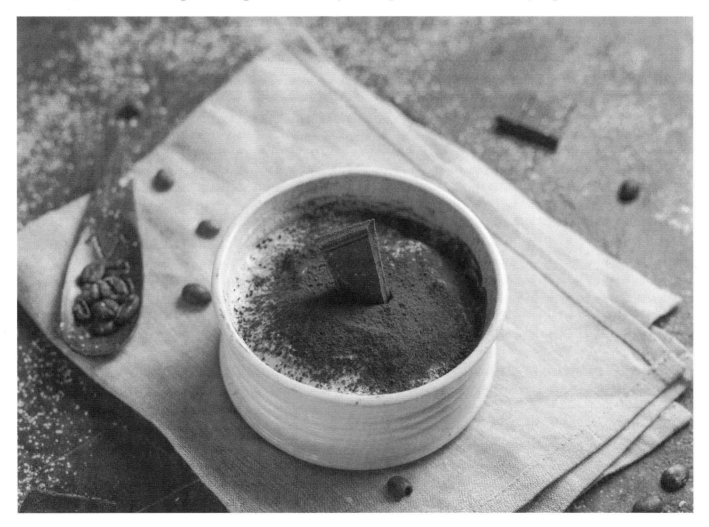

51. Coconut Lime Protein Balls

Prep: 10 minutes   Cook: None (chill for 30 minutes)   Serves: 6

INGREDIENTS

- 1 cup shredded unsweetened coconut
- 2 scoops vanilla protein powder
- 2 tablespoons coconut oil, melted
- Zest and juice of 1 lime
- 1 tablespoon honey or low-carb sweetener

INSTRUCTIONS

1. In a bowl, mix shredded coconut, protein powder, coconut oil, lime zest, lime juice, and honey.
2. Form into small balls and place them in the fridge for at least 30 minutes to firm up.
3. Serve chilled.

Nutritional Facts (Per Serving):
Calories: 160 **Fat**: 12g **Carbohydrates**: 5g **Protein**: 10g

52. Coconut Almond Protein Bites

Prep: 10 minutes   Cook: None (chill for 30 minutes)   Serves: 6

INGREDIENTS

- 1 cup almond flour
- 2 scoops vanilla protein powder
- ¼ cup almond butter
- 1 tablespoon honey or low-carb sweetener
- ¼ cup shredded unsweetened coconut

INSTRUCTIONS

1. In a bowl, mix almond flour, protein powder, almond butter, honey, and shredded coconut.
2. Roll the mixture into small balls and refrigerate for at least 30 minutes to set.
3. Serve chilled or at room temperature.

Nutritional Facts (Per Serving):
Calories: 180 **Fat**: 14g **Carbohydrates**: 5g **Protein**: 10g

53. Chocolate Protein Pudding

Prep: 5 minutes   **Cook: None (chill for 30 minutes)**   **Serves: 2**

INGREDIENTS

- 2 scoops chocolate protein powder
- 1 cup unsweetened almond milk
- 1 tablespoon cocoa powder
- 1 teaspoon vanilla extract
- 1 tablespoon chia seeds (optional)

INSTRUCTIONS

1. In a blender, combine protein powder, almond milk, cocoa powder, and vanilla extract. Blend until smooth.
2. Stir in chia seeds if desired for extra thickness, then refrigerate for 30 minutes to set.
3. Serve chilled.

Nutritional Facts (Per Serving):
Calories: 200 **Fat**: 6g **Carbohydrates**: 8g **Protein**: 25g

54. Lemon Raspberry Protein Bars

Prep: 10 minutes   **Cook: None (chill for 1 hour)**   **Serves: 6**

INGREDIENTS

- 2 scoops vanilla protein powder
- 1 cup almond flour
- ¼ cup fresh raspberries
- Zest and juice of 1 lemon
- 1 tablespoon coconut oil, melted

INSTRUCTIONS

1. In a bowl, combine protein powder, almond flour, lemon zest, lemon juice, and coconut oil.
2. Gently fold in raspberries.
3. Press the mixture into a parchment-lined dish and refrigerate for 1 hour to set.
4. Cut into bars and serve chilled.

Nutritional Facts (Per Serving):
Calories: 180 **Fat**: 12g **Carbohydrates**: 7g **Protein**: 15g

55. Pumpkin Protein Muffins

| Prep: 10 minutes | Cook: 20 minutes | Serves: 6 |

INGREDIENTS

- ½ cup canned pumpkin
- 2 scoops vanilla protein powder
- ¼ cup almond flour
- 2 large eggs
- 1 teaspoon baking powder
- 1 teaspoon pumpkin spice
- 2 tablespoons coconut oil, melted

INSTRUCTIONS

1. Preheat the oven to 350°F (175°C). Grease a muffin tin.
2. In a bowl, mix pumpkin, protein powder, almond flour, eggs, baking powder, pumpkin spice, and coconut oil until well combined.
3. Divide the batter evenly into the muffin tin and bake for 18-20 minutes or until a toothpick comes out clean.
4. Let cool and serve.

Nutritional Facts (Per Serving):
Calories: 150 **Fat**: 10g **Carbohydrates**: 5g **Protein**: 12g

56. Strawberry Protein Cheesecake

| Prep: 10 minutes | Cook: None (chill for 1 hour) | Serves: 4 |

INGREDIENTS

- 1 cup low-fat cream cheese
- 2 scoops vanilla protein powder
- ½ cup fresh strawberries, mashed
- 1 tablespoon honey or low-carb sweetener
- 1 teaspoon vanilla extract

INSTRUCTIONS

1. In a bowl, mix cream cheese, protein powder, mashed strawberries, honey, and vanilla extract until smooth.
2. Spoon into small serving cups and refrigerate for 1 hour to set.
3. Serve chilled.

Nutritional Facts (Per Serving):
Calories: 180 **Fat**: 12g **Carbohydrates**: 6g **Protein**: 12g

57. Peanut Butter Cookies

| Prep: 10 minutes | Cook: 10 minutes | Serves: 8 |

INGREDIENTS

- 1 cup natural peanut butter
- 2 scoops vanilla or chocolate protein powder
- 1 large egg
- 1 teaspoon baking powder
- 1 tablespoon honey or low-carb sweetener

INSTRUCTIONS

1. Preheat the oven to 350°F (175°C) and line a baking sheet with parchment paper.
2. In a bowl, mix peanut butter, protein powder, egg, baking powder, and honey until combined.
3. Scoop dough into small balls, place on the baking sheet, and flatten with a fork.
4. Bake for 10 minutes or until golden. Let cool before serving.

Nutritional Facts (Per Serving):
Calories: 200 **Fat:** 15g **Carbohydrates:** 6g **Protein:** 12g

58. Mocha Mousse

| Prep: 5 minutes | Cook: None (chill for 30 minutes) | Serves: 2 |

INGREDIENTS

- 2 scoops chocolate protein powder
- 1 cup unsweetened almond milk
- 1 tablespoon instant coffee granules
- 1 tablespoon cocoa powder
- 1 tablespoon chia seeds (optional)

INSTRUCTIONS

1. Blend protein powder, almond milk, coffee granules, and cocoa powder until smooth.
2. Stir in chia seeds for thickness, then refrigerate for 30 minutes.
3. Serve chilled.

Nutritional Facts (Per Serving):
Calories: 180 **Fat:** 5g **Carbohydrates:** 6g **Protein:** 25g

59. Chocolate Chip Cookies

Prep: 10 minutes	Cook: 10 minutes	Serves: 8

INGREDIENTS

- 1 cup almond flour
- 2 scoops vanilla protein powder
- ¼ cup sugar-free chocolate chips
- 1 large egg
- 1 tablespoon coconut oil, melted
- 1 teaspoon vanilla extract

INSTRUCTIONS

1. Preheat the oven to 350°F (175°C) and line a baking sheet with parchment paper.
2. In a bowl, mix almond flour, protein powder, egg, coconut oil, and vanilla extract until combined.
3. Fold in the chocolate chips, scoop dough onto the baking sheet, and flatten each cookie slightly.
4. Bake for 10 minutes or until golden. Let cool before serving.

Nutritional Facts (Per Serving):
Calories: 180 **Fat:** 12g **Carbohydrates:** 6g **Protein:** 10g

60. Matcha Latte

Prep: 5 minutes	Cook: None	Serves: 1

INGREDIENTS

- 1 teaspoon matcha green tea powder
- 1 cup unsweetened almond milk
- 1 scoop vanilla protein powder
- 1 teaspoon honey or low-carb sweetener (optional)

INSTRUCTIONS

1. In a blender, mix almond milk, protein powder, matcha, and sweetener until smooth and frothy.
2. Serve immediately over ice or warm it up for a hot matcha latte.

Nutritional Facts (Per Serving):
Calories: 150 **Fat:** 5g **Carbohydrates:** 8g **Protein:** 15g

61. Coconut Protein Truffles

Prep: 10 minutes   **Cook: None (chill for 30 minutes)**   **Serves: 6**

INGREDIENTS

- 1 cup shredded unsweetened coconut
- 2 scoops vanilla protein powder
- 2 tablespoons coconut oil, melted
- 1 tablespoon honey or low-carb sweetener
- ½ teaspoon vanilla extract

INSTRUCTIONS

1. Mix all the ingredients in a bowl until well combined.
2. Form into small balls and refrigerate for 30 minutes to firm up.
3. Serve chilled.

Nutritional Facts (Per Serving):
Calories: 180 **Fat:** 14g **Carbohydrates:** 5g **Protein:** 10g

62. Apple Cinnamon Muffins

Prep: 10 minutes   **Cook: 20 minutes**   **Serves: 6**

INGREDIENTS

- 1 cup almond flour
- 2 scoops vanilla protein powder
- 1 large apple, grated
- 1 teaspoon cinnamon
- 1 large egg
- 1 tablespoon honey or low-carb sweetener
- 1 teaspoon baking powder

INSTRUCTIONS

1. Preheat the oven to 350°F (175°C) and grease a muffin tin.
2. In a bowl, mix almond flour, protein powder, cinnamon, egg, honey, and baking powder.
3. Stir in the grated apple.
4. Divide the batter into the muffin tin and bake for 18-20 minutes, or until a toothpick comes out clean.
5. Let cool before serving.

Nutritional Facts (Per Serving):
Calories: 180 **Fat:** 10g **Carbohydrates:** 12g **Protein:** 12g

63. Chocolate Mint Protein Bars

Prep: 10 minutes   **Cook: None (chill for 1 hour)**   **Serves: 6**

INGREDIENTS

- 2 scoops chocolate protein powder
- 1 cup almond flour
- 1 teaspoon peppermint extract
- ¼ cup dark chocolate chips (sugar-free)
- 2 tablespoons coconut oil, melted

INSTRUCTIONS

1. In a bowl, combine protein powder, almond flour, peppermint extract, and coconut oil.
2. Fold in the dark chocolate chips.
3. Press the mixture into a parchment-lined dish and refrigerate for 1 hour to set.
4. Cut into bars and serve.

Nutritional Facts (Per Serving):
Calories: 180 **Fat:** 12g **Carbohydrates:** 5g **Protein:** 12g

64. Vanilla Ice Cream

Prep: 5 minutes   **Cook: None (freeze for 1 hour)**   **Serves: 4**

INGREDIENTS

- 2 cups full-fat coconut milk
- 2 scoops vanilla protein powder
- 1 teaspoon vanilla extract
- 1 tablespoon honey or low-carb sweetener

INSTRUCTIONS

1. In a blender, combine coconut milk, protein powder, vanilla extract, and honey until smooth.
2. Pour the mixture into a shallow dish and freeze for at least 1 hour.
3. Scoop and serve.

Nutritional Facts (Per Serving):
Calories: 150 **Fat:** 12g **Carbohydrates:** 5g **Protein:** 10g

65. Vanilla Almond Protein Balls

Prep: 10 minutes	Cook: None (chill for 30 minutes)	Serves: 6

INGREDIENTS

- 1 cup almond flour
- 2 scoops vanilla protein powder
- ¼ cup almond butter
- 1 teaspoon vanilla extract
- 1 tablespoon honey or low-carb sweetener

INSTRUCTIONS

1. In a bowl, mix almond flour, protein powder, almond butter, vanilla extract, and honey until combined.
2. Roll into small balls and refrigerate for 30 minutes.
3. Serve chilled.

Nutritional Facts (Per Serving):
Calories: 190 **Fat**: 12g **Carbohydrates**: 5g **Protein**: 10g

66. Berry Gelatin

Prep: 5 minutes	Cook: None (chill for 2 hours)	Serves: 4

INGREDIENTS

- 1 cup mixed berries (strawberries, blueberries, raspberries)
- 1 packet sugar-free gelatin mix
- 2 cups water

INSTRUCTIONS

1. Prepare the gelatin according to the package instructions.
2. Divide the mixed berries between serving cups and pour the prepared gelatin over them.
3. Refrigerate for 2 hours until set. Serve chilled.

Nutritional Facts (Per Serving):
Calories: 50 **Fat**: 0g **Carbohydrates**: 7g **Protein**: 5g

67. Peanut Butter Cups

Prep: 10 minutes	Cook: None (chill for 30 minutes)	Serves: 6

INGREDIENTS

- 1 cup natural peanut butter
- ½ cup sugar-free dark chocolate chips
- 2 tablespoons coconut oil

INSTRUCTIONS

1. Melt the chocolate chips and coconut oil in a microwave-safe bowl.
2. Pour a small amount of melted chocolate into the bottom of silicone muffin cups.
3. Add a spoonful of peanut butter on top, then cover with more melted chocolate.
4. Refrigerate for 30 minutes until set. Serve chilled.

Nutritional Facts (Per Serving):
Calories: 200 **Fat:** 16g **Carbohydrates:** 7g **Protein:** 8g

68. Cinnamon Roll Bites

Prep: 10 minutes	Cook: None (chill for 30 minutes)	Serves: 6

INGREDIENTS

- 1 cup almond flour
- 2 scoops vanilla protein powder
- 1 tablespoon cinnamon
- ¼ cup almond butter
- 1 tablespoon honey or low-carb sweetener

INSTRUCTIONS

1. Mix almond flour, protein powder, cinnamon, almond butter, and honey in a bowl.
2. Form into small balls and refrigerate for 30 minutes to firm up.
3. Serve chilled.

Nutritional Facts (Per Serving):
Calories: 180 **Fat:** 12g **Carbohydrates:** 6g **Protein:** 12g

69. Chocolate Banana Bread

Prep: 10 minutes	Cook: 30 minutes	Serves: 6

INGREDIENTS

- 1 cup almond flour
- 2 scoops chocolate protein powder
- 1 ripe banana, mashed
- 2 large eggs
- 1 tablespoon cocoa powder
- 1 teaspoon baking powder

INSTRUCTIONS

1. Preheat the oven to 350°F (175°C) and grease a loaf pan.
2. In a bowl, mix almond flour, protein powder, mashed banana, eggs, cocoa powder, and baking powder.
3. Pour the batter into the pan and bake for 25-30 minutes, or until a toothpick comes out clean.
4. Let cool before serving.

Nutritional Facts (Per Serving):
Calories: 180 **Fat**: 8g **Carbohydrates**: 12g **Protein**: 12g

70. Chocolate Coconut Bars

Prep: 10 minutes	Cook: None (chill for 1 hour)	Serves: 6

INGREDIENTS

- 1 cup shredded unsweetened coconut
- 2 scoops chocolate protein powder
- ¼ cup coconut oil, melted
- 1 tablespoon honey or low-carb sweetener

INSTRUCTIONS

1. In a bowl, combine shredded coconut, protein powder, coconut oil, and honey.
2. Press the mixture into a parchment-lined dish and refrigerate for 1 hour to set.
3. Cut into bars and serve.

Nutritional Facts (Per Serving):
Calories: 200 **Fat**: 16g **Carbohydrates**: 6g **Protein**: 10g

71. Protein Cheesecake Bites

Prep: 10 minutes   Cook: None (chill for 1 hour)   Serves: 6

INGREDIENTS

- 1 cup low-fat cream cheese
- 2 scoops vanilla protein powder
- 1 tablespoon honey or low-carb sweetener
- 1 teaspoon vanilla extract

INSTRUCTIONS

1. In a bowl, mix cream cheese, protein powder, honey, and vanilla extract until smooth.
2. Spoon the mixture into silicone muffin cups and refrigerate for 1 hour to set.
3. Serve chilled.

Nutritional Facts (Per Serving):
Calories: 150 **Fat**: 10g **Carbohydrates**: 4g **Protein**: 12g

72. Almond Flour Cookies

Prep: 10 minutes   Cook: 10 minutes   Serves: 8

INGREDIENTS

- 1 cup almond flour
- 2 scoops vanilla protein powder
- 1 large egg
- 1 tablespoon coconut oil, melted
- 1 teaspoon vanilla extract

INSTRUCTIONS

1. Preheat the oven to 350°F (175°C) and line a baking sheet with parchment paper.
2. In a bowl, mix almond flour, protein powder, egg, coconut oil, and vanilla extract until combined.
3. Scoop dough onto the baking sheet and flatten each cookie slightly.
4. Bake for 10 minutes or until golden. Let cool before serving.

Nutritional Facts (Per Serving):
Calories: 180 **Fat**: 12g **Carbohydrates**: 5g **Protein**: 10g

73. Avocado Brownies

Prep: 10 minutes   **Cook: 25 minutes**   **Serves: 6**

INGREDIENTS

- 1 ripe avocado, mashed
- ½ cup cocoa powder
- 2 scoops chocolate protein powder
- 1 tablespoon coconut oil, melted
- 2 large eggs
- 1 teaspoon vanilla extract

INSTRUCTIONS

1. Preheat the oven to 350°F (175°C) and grease a baking dish.
2. In a bowl, mix mashed avocado, cocoa powder, protein powder, coconut oil, eggs, and vanilla extract until smooth.
3. Pour the batter into the baking dish and bake for 20-25 minutes.
4. Let cool before serving.

Nutritional Facts (Per Serving):
Calories: 180 **Fat:** 12g **Carbohydrates:** 7g **Protein:** 12g

74. Carrot Cake

Prep: 10 minutes   **Cook: 30 minutes**   **Serves: 6**

INGREDIENTS

- 1 cup almond flour
- 2 scoops vanilla protein powder
- 1 large carrot, grated
- 2 large eggs
- 1 teaspoon cinnamon
- 1 tablespoon coconut oil, melted
- 1 teaspoon baking powder

INSTRUCTIONS

1. Preheat the oven to 350°F (175°C) and grease a loaf pan.
2. In a bowl, mix almond flour, protein powder, grated carrot, eggs, cinnamon, coconut oil, and baking powder.
3. Pour the batter into the pan and bake for 25-30 minutes, or until a toothpick comes out clean.
4. Let cool before serving.

Nutritional Facts (Per Serving):
Calories: 190 **Fat:** 10g **Carbohydrates:** 10g **Protein:** 12g

75. Protein Cupcakes

Prep: 10 minutes   **Cook: 20 minutes**   **Serves: 6**

INGREDIENTS

- 1 cup almond flour
- 2 scoops vanilla protein powder
- 2 large eggs
- 1 tablespoon coconut oil, melted
- 1 teaspoon vanilla extract
- 1 teaspoon baking powder

INSTRUCTIONS

1. Preheat the oven to 350°F (175°C) and line a muffin tin with paper cups.
2. In a bowl, mix almond flour, protein powder, eggs, coconut oil, vanilla extract, and baking powder until combined.
3. Divide the batter into the muffin tin and bake for 18-20 minutes or until a toothpick comes out clean.
4. Let cool before serving.

Nutritional Facts (Per Serving):
Calories: 180 **Fat:** 12g **Carbohydrates:** 5g **Protein:** 12g

CHAPTER 7

Smoothies and Protein Drinks: Fuel for Your Day

Smoothies and protein drinks are the perfect way to refuel after a workout, boost your morning, or provide a quick and nutritious snack during the day. Packed with protein, healthy fats, and nutrient-dense fruits and veggies, these drinks are not only delicious but also keep you energized for hours.

This chapter is filled with 25 refreshing smoothie and protein drink recipes that are easy to make and tailored to fit a low-carb, high-protein lifestyle. Whether you need a green smoothie for a quick health boost or a creamy chocolate protein shake to satisfy your sweet tooth, these recipes are versatile and perfect for any time of day.

Let's get blending!

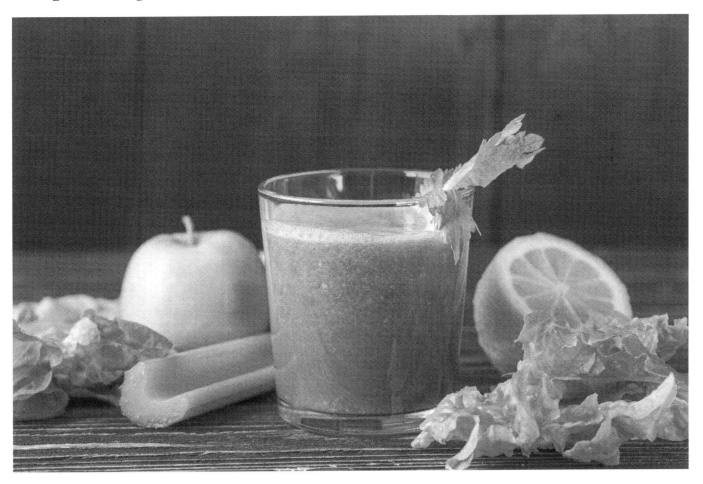

76. Berry Almond Smoothie

| Prep: 5 minutes | Cook: None | Serves: 1 |

INGREDIENTS

- 1 cup unsweetened almond milk
- ½ cup mixed berries (strawberries, blueberries, raspberries)
- 1 tablespoon almond butter
- 1 scoop vanilla protein powder
- 1 teaspoon chia seeds (optional)

INSTRUCTIONS

1. Blend almond milk, berries, almond butter, and protein powder until smooth.
2. Add chia seeds if desired for extra fiber and blend again.
3. Serve immediately.

Nutritional Facts (Per Serving):
Calories: 220 **Fat**: 12g **Carbohydrates**: 12g **Protein**: 18g

77. Peanut Butter Banana Smoothie

| Prep: 5 minutes | Cook: None | Serves: 1 |

INGREDIENTS

- 1 cup unsweetened almond milk
- 1 tablespoon peanut butter
- ½ banana, frozen
- 1 scoop vanilla protein powder

INSTRUCTIONS

1. Blend almond milk, peanut butter, banana, and protein powder until smooth.
2. Serve immediately.

Nutritional Facts (Per Serving):
Calories: 240 **Fat**: 10g **Carbohydrates**: 18g **Protein**: 20g

78. Greek Yogurt Berry Smoothie

Prep: 5 minutes	Cook: None	Serves: 1

INGREDIENTS

- ½ cup plain Greek yogurt
- 1 cup mixed berries (strawberries, blueberries, raspberries)
- ½ cup unsweetened almond milk
- 1 scoop vanilla protein powder

INSTRUCTIONS

1. Blend Greek yogurt, berries, almond milk, and protein powder until smooth.
2. Serve immediately.

Nutritional Facts (Per Serving):
Calories: 220 **Fat**: 5g **Carbohydrates**: 18g **Protein**: 25g

79. Green Protein Smoothie

Prep: 5 minutes	Cook: None	Serves: 1

INGREDIENTS

- 1 cup spinach
- 1 small cucumber, chopped
- 1 green apple, chopped
- 1 scoop vanilla protein powder
- 1 cup water

INSTRUCTIONS

1. Blend spinach, cucumber, apple, protein powder, and water until smooth.
2. Serve immediately.

Nutritional Facts (Per Serving):
Calories: 160 **Fat**: 2g **Carbohydrates**: 22g **Protein**: 15g

80. Chocolate Banana Smoothie

Prep: 5 minutes   Cook: None   Serves: 1

INGREDIENTS

- 1 cup unsweetened almond milk
- 1 scoop chocolate protein powder
- ½ banana, frozen
- 1 tablespoon cocoa powder

INSTRUCTIONS

1. Blend almond milk, protein powder, banana, and cocoa powder until smooth.
2. Serve immediately.

Nutritional Facts (Per Serving):
Calories: 230 **Fat:** 8g **Carbohydrates:** 22g **Protein:** 20g

81. Coconut Mango Smoothie

Prep: 5 minutes   Cook: None   Serves: 1

INGREDIENTS

- 1 cup unsweetened coconut milk
- ½ cup frozen mango chunks
- 1 scoop vanilla protein powder
- 1 tablespoon shredded unsweetened coconut

INSTRUCTIONS

1. Blend coconut milk, mango, protein powder, and shredded coconut until smooth.
2. Serve immediately.

Nutritional Facts (Per Serving):
Calories: 250 **Fat:** 12g **Carbohydrates:** 20g **Protein:** 18g

82. Broccoli Apple Smoothie

| Prep: 5 minutes | Cook: None | Serves: 1 |

INGREDIENTS

- 1 small apple, chopped
- 1 cup broccoli florets (blanched)
- 1 scoop vanilla protein powder
- 1 cup water

INSTRUCTIONS

1. Blend apple, broccoli, protein powder, and water until smooth.
2. Serve immediately.

Nutritional Facts (Per Serving):
Calories: 160 **Fat**: 2g **Carbohydrates**: 22g **Protein**: 15g

83. Vanilla Blueberry Smoothie

| Prep: 5 minutes | Cook: None | Serves: 1 |

INGREDIENTS

- 1 cup unsweetened almond milk
- ½ cup blueberries, frozen
- 1 scoop vanilla protein powder
- 1 teaspoon chia seeds (optional)

INSTRUCTIONS

1. Blend almond milk, blueberries, protein powder, and chia seeds until smooth.
2. Serve immediately.

Nutritional Facts (Per Serving):
Calories: 180 **Fat**: 6g **Carbohydrates**: 15g **Protein**: 18g

84. Peanut Butter Cup Smoothie

Prep: 5 minutes   Cook: None   Serves: 1

INGREDIENTS

- 1 cup unsweetened almond milk
- 1 tablespoon peanut butter
- 1 scoop chocolate protein powder
- 1 teaspoon cocoa powder

INSTRUCTIONS

1. Blend almond milk, peanut butter, protein powder, and cocoa powder until smooth.
2. Serve immediately.

Nutritional Facts (Per Serving):
Calories: 240 **Fat**: 12g **Carbohydrates**: 8g **Protein**: 20g

85. Blueberry Almond Smoothie

Prep: 5 minutes   Cook: None   Serves: 1

INGREDIENTS

- 1 cup unsweetened almond milk
- ½ cup frozen blueberries
- 1 tablespoon almond butter
- 1 scoop vanilla protein powder

INSTRUCTIONS

1. Blend almond milk, blueberries, almond butter, and protein powder until smooth.
2. Serve immediately.

Nutritional Facts (Per Serving):
Calories: 210 **Fat**: 12g **Carbohydrates**: 14g **Protein**: 18g

86. Chocolate Hazelnut Smoothie

Prep: 5 minutes	Cook: None	Serves: 1

INGREDIENTS

- 1 cup unsweetened almond milk
- 1 tablespoon hazelnut butter
- 1 scoop chocolate protein powder
- 1 tablespoon cocoa powder

INSTRUCTIONS

1. Blend almond milk, hazelnut butter, protein powder, and cocoa powder until smooth.
2. Serve immediately.

Nutritional Facts (Per Serving):
Calories: 230 **Fat**: 14g **Carbohydrates**: 8g **Protein**: 18g

87. Chocolate Cherry Smoothie

Prep: 5 minutes	Cook: None	Serves: 1

INGREDIENTS

- 1 cup unsweetened almond milk
- ½ cup frozen cherries
- 1 scoop chocolate protein powder
- 1 tablespoon cocoa powder

INSTRUCTIONS

1. Blend almond milk, cherries, protein powder, and cocoa powder until smooth.
2. Serve immediately.

Nutritional Facts (Per Serving):
Calories: 220 **Fat**: 8g **Carbohydrates**: 22g **Protein**: 18g

88. Carrot Ginger Smoothie

Prep: 5 minutes   Cook: None   Serves: 1

INGREDIENTS

- 1 small carrot, peeled and chopped
- 1 teaspoon fresh ginger, grated
- 1 cup unsweetened almond milk
- 1 scoop vanilla protein powder

INSTRUCTIONS

1. Blend carrot, ginger, almond milk, and protein powder until smooth.
2. Serve immediately.

Nutritional Facts (Per Serving):
Calories: 160 **Fat:** 5g **Carbohydrates:** 10g **Protein:** 15g

89. Pumpkin Spice Smoothie

Prep: 5 minutes   Cook: None   Serves: 1

INGREDIENTS

- ½ cup canned pumpkin
- 1 cup unsweetened almond milk
- 1 scoop vanilla protein powder
- ½ teaspoon pumpkin spice
- 1 teaspoon honey or low-carb sweetener (optional)

INSTRUCTIONS

1. Blend pumpkin, almond milk, protein powder, pumpkin spice, and honey until smooth.
2. Serve immediately.

Nutritional Facts (Per Serving):
Calories: 170 **Fat:** 6g **Carbohydrates:** 12g **Protein:** 18g

90. Strawberry Avocado Smoothie

| Prep: 5 minutes | Cook: None | Serves: 1 |

INGREDIENTS

- 1 small avocado
- 1 cup strawberries, frozen
- 1 cup unsweetened almond milk
- 1 scoop vanilla protein powder

INSTRUCTIONS

1. Blend avocado, strawberries, almond milk, and protein powder until smooth.
2. Serve immediately.

Nutritional Facts (Per Serving):
Calories: 250 **Fat:** 14g **Carbohydrates:** 15g **Protein:** 18g

91. Mocha Protein Smoothie

| Prep: 5 minutes | Cook: None | Serves: 1 |

INGREDIENTS

- 1 cup unsweetened almond milk
- 1 scoop chocolate protein powder
- 1 tablespoon cocoa powder
- 1 teaspoon instant coffee granules

INSTRUCTIONS

1. Blend almond milk, protein powder, cocoa powder, and coffee granules until smooth.
2. Serve immediately.

Nutritional Facts (Per Serving):
Calories: 210 **Fat:** 8g **Carbohydrates:** 6g **Protein:** 18g

92. Lemon Blueberry Smoothie

Prep: 5 minutes   Cook: None   Serves: 1

INGREDIENTS

- 1 cup unsweetened almond milk
- ½ cup blueberries, frozen
- Zest and juice of 1 lemon
- 1 scoop vanilla protein powder

INSTRUCTIONS

1. Blend almond milk, blueberries, lemon zest, lemon juice, and protein powder until smooth.
2. Serve immediately.

Nutritional Facts (Per Serving):
Calories: 180 **Fat**: 6g **Carbohydrates**: 15g **Protein**: 18g

93. Tomato Basil Smoothie

Prep: 5 minutes   Cook: None   Serves: 1

INGREDIENTS

- 1 medium tomato, chopped
- 1 cup unsweetened almond milk
- 1 scoop vanilla protein powder
- 5 fresh basil leaves
- Salt and pepper to taste

INSTRUCTIONS

1. Blend tomato, almond milk, protein powder, basil, salt, and pepper until smooth.
2. Serve immediately.

Nutritional Facts (Per Serving):
Calories: 150 **Fat**: 5g **Carbohydrates**: 10g **Protein**: 18g

94. Mint Chocolate Smoothie

Prep: 5 minutes   **Cook: None**   **Serves: 1**

INGREDIENTS

- 1 cup unsweetened almond milk
- 1 tablespoon fresh mint leaves
- 1 scoop chocolate protein powder
- 1 tablespoon cocoa powder

INSTRUCTIONS

1. Blend almond milk, mint leaves, protein powder, and cocoa powder until smooth.
2. Serve immediately.

Nutritional Facts (Per Serving):
Calories: 190 **Fat**: 8g **Carbohydrates**: 7g **Protein**: 18g

95. Raspberry Coconut Smoothie

Prep: 5 minutes   **Cook: None**   **Serves: 1**

INGREDIENTS

- 1 cup unsweetened coconut milk
- ½ cup raspberries, frozen
- 1 scoop vanilla protein powder
- 1 tablespoon shredded unsweetened coconut

INSTRUCTIONS

1. Blend coconut milk, raspberries, protein powder, and shredded coconut until smooth.
2. Serve immediately.

Nutritional Facts (Per Serving):
Calories: 210 **Fat**: 12g **Carbohydrates**: 12g **Protein**: 18g

96. Peach Smoothie

Prep: 5 minutes   Cook: None   Serves: 1

INGREDIENTS

- 1 cup unsweetened almond milk
- 1 large peach, chopped
- 1 scoop vanilla protein powder
- 1 tablespoon chia seeds (optional)

INSTRUCTIONS

1. Blend almond milk, peach, protein powder, and chia seeds until smooth.
2. Serve immediately.

Nutritional Facts (Per Serving):
Calories: 190 **Fat:** 5g **Carbohydrates:** 20g **Protein:** 18g

97. Spinach Smoothie

Prep: 5 minutes   Cook: None   Serves: 1

INGREDIENTS

- 1 cup spinach
- 1 small cucumber, chopped
- 1 green apple, chopped
- 1 scoop vanilla protein powder
- 1 cup water

INSTRUCTIONS

1. Blend spinach, cucumber, apple, protein powder, and water until smooth.
2. Serve immediately.

Nutritional Facts (Per Serving):
Calories: 160 **Fat:** 2g **Carbohydrates:** 22g **Protein:** 15g

98. Citrus Ginger Detox Infusion

Prep: 5 minutes   **Cook: None**   **Serves: 1**

INGREDIENTS

- 1 small orange, peeled
- 1 lemon, peeled
- 1 teaspoon fresh ginger, grated
- 1 cup cold water

INSTRUCTIONS

1. Blend orange, lemon, ginger, and water until smooth.
2. Serve immediately or over ice.

Nutritional Facts (Per Serving):
Calories: 60 **Fat**: 0g **Carbohydrates**: 15g **Protein**: 1g

99. Avocado Smoothie

Prep: 5 minutes   **Cook: None**   **Serves: 1**

INGREDIENTS

- 1 small avocado
- 1 cup unsweetened almond milk
- 1 scoop vanilla protein powder
- 1 teaspoon honey or low-carb sweetener (optional)

INSTRUCTIONS

1. Blend avocado, almond milk, protein powder, and honey until smooth.
2. Serve immediately.

Nutritional Facts (Per Serving):
Calories: 250 **Fat**: 14g **Carbohydrates**: 12g **Protein**: 18g

100. Mango Smoothie

| Prep: 5 minutes | Cook: None | Serves: 1 |

INGREDIENTS

- 1 cup unsweetened almond milk
- ½ cup frozen mango chunks
- 1 scoop vanilla protein powder
- 1 tablespoon chia seeds (optional)

INSTRUCTIONS

1. Blend almond milk, mango, protein powder, and chia seeds until smooth.
2. Serve immediately.

Nutritional Facts (Per Serving):
Calories: 190 **Fat:** 6g **Carbohydrates:** 22g **Protein:** 18g

PART 3

MEAL PLANS AND BONUS CONTENT

CHAPTER 8

Your 28-Day Jumpstart: The First Four Weeks

The first four weeks of any lifestyle change are critical. This is the period where you build new habits, reset your body, and lay the foundation for long-term success. The 28-Day Jumpstart is designed to help you kick off your low-carb, high-protein journey with focus and clarity. The goal is to fuel your body with nutritious, protein-packed meals while controlling carbohydrates, which will help you feel more energized, control cravings, and begin to see weight loss and muscle toning results.

This plan is structured around four core phases, each lasting one week. As you progress through each week, you'll notice a gradual shift in your energy levels, how you feel about your food choices, and, most importantly, how your body responds. These meals are all taken from the recipes in this book, providing a variety of flavors and textures while keeping you on track.

Week 1: Detox and Protein Boost

DAY	BREAKFAST	LUNCH	DINNER
Day 1	1. Greek Yogurt Parfait with Berries & Nuts	16. Grilled Chicken Caesar Salad	31. Grilled Steak with Chimichurri Sauce
Day 2	2. Spinach & Feta Omelette	17. Turkey Avocado Wrap	32. Baked Lemon Herb Salmon
Day 3	3. Avocado & Smoked Salmon Toast	18. Baked Salmon with Dill & Lemon	33. Balsamic Glazed Chicken
Day 4	4. Cottage Cheese with Berries & Almonds	19. Eggplant Lasagna	34. Lemon Garlic Shrimp Pasta
Day 5	5. Scrambled Eggs with Spinach & Tomatoes	20. Shrimp & Avocado Salad	35. Pesto Zoodles with Chicken
Day 6	6. Chia Seed Pudding with Almond Milk & Berries	21. Grilled Chicken & Pesto Wrap	36. Garlic Butter Shrimp with Asparagus
Day 7	7. Egg Muffins	22. Chicken & Vegetable Skewers	37. Lamb Chops with Mint Yogurt Sauce

Week 2: Building Healthy Habits

DAY	BREAKFAST	LUNCH	DINNER
Day 8	1. Greek Yogurt Parfait with Berries & Nuts	16. Grilled Chicken Caesar Salad	31. Grilled Steak with Chimichurri Sauce
Day 9	2. Spinach & Feta Omelette	17. Turkey Avocado Wrap	32. Baked Lemon Herb Salmon
Day 10	3. Avocado & Smoked Salmon Toast	18. Baked Salmon with Dill & Lemon	33. Balsamic Glazed Chicken
Day 11	4. Cottage Cheese with Berries & Almonds	19. Eggplant Lasagna	34. Lemon Garlic Shrimp Pasta
Day 12	5. Scrambled Eggs with Spinach & Tomatoes	20. Shrimp & Avocado Salad	35. Pesto Zoodles with Chicken
Day 13	6. Chia Seed Pudding with Almond Milk & Berries	21. Grilled Chicken & Pesto Wrap	36. Garlic Butter Shrimp with Asparagus
Day 14	7. Egg Muffins	22. Chicken & Vegetable Skewers	37. Lamb Chops with Mint Yogurt Sauce

Week 3: Muscle Toning with Protein Variations

DAY	BREAKFAST	LUNCH	DINNER
Day 15	1. Greek Yogurt Parfait with Berries & Nuts	16. Grilled Chicken Caesar Salad	31. Grilled Steak with Chimichurri Sauce
Day 16	2. Spinach & Feta Omelette	17. Turkey Avocado Wrap	32. Baked Lemon Herb Salmon
Day 17	3. Avocado & Smoked Salmon Toast	18. Baked Salmon with Dill & Lemon	33. Balsamic Glazed Chicken
Day 18	4. Cottage Cheese with Berries & Almonds	19. Eggplant Lasagna	34. Lemon Garlic Shrimp Pasta
Day 19	5. Scrambled Eggs with Spinach & Tomatoes	20. Shrimp & Avocado Salad	35. Pesto Zoodles with Chicken
Day 20	6. Chia Seed Pudding with Almond Milk & Berries	21. Grilled Chicken & Pesto Wrap	36. Garlic Butter Shrimp with Asparagus

| Day 21 | 7. Egg Muffins | 22. Chicken & Vegetable Skewers | 37. Lamb Chops with Mint Yogurt Sauce |

Week 4: Portion Control and Maintenance

DAY	BREAKFAST	LUNCH	DINNER
Day 22	1. Greek Yogurt Parfait with Berries & Nuts	16. Grilled Chicken Caesar Salad	31. Grilled Steak with Chimichurri Sauce
Day 23	2. Spinach & Feta Omelette	17. Turkey Avocado Wrap	32. Baked Lemon Herb Salmon
Day 24	3. Avocado & Smoked Salmon Toast	18. Baked Salmon with Dill & Lemon	33. Balsamic Glazed Chicken
Day 25	4. Cottage Cheese with Berries & Almonds	19. Eggplant Lasagna	34. Lemon Garlic Shrimp Pasta
Day 26	5. Scrambled Eggs with Spinach & Tomatoes	20. Shrimp & Avocado Salad	35. Pesto Zoodles with Chicken
Day 27	6. Chia Seed Pudding with Almond Milk & Berries	21. Grilled Chicken & Pesto Wrap	36. Garlic Butter Shrimp with Asparagus
Day 28	7. Egg Muffins	22. Chicken & Vegetable Skewers	37. Lamb Chops with Mint Yogurt Sauce

CHAPTER 9

The Complete 60-Day Meal Plan: Sustainable Results

After completing the 28-Day Jumpstart, your body is primed for continued progress. You've established new habits, started to see results, and feel more energized. Now, it's time to take it to the next level with a comprehensive 60-day meal plan designed to bring sustainable results. This phase of the program will guide you through an additional nine weeks of low-carb, high-protein meals, with a focus on maintaining or accelerating weight loss, building muscle, and refining your portion control.

This meal plan is not a one-size-fits-all approach. While it includes a wide variety of delicious and nutritious meals, it also offers flexibility, allowing you to tailor your meals depending on your personal goals. Whether you're looking to shed those extra pounds or build lean muscle, this 60-day plan provides a structured yet adaptable guide.

The plan is divided into three main phases, each lasting three weeks. By following these detailed meal plans for breakfast, lunch, and dinner, you'll develop a routine that's sustainable and fits your lifestyle, helping you achieve long-term success.

Weeks 1-3: Maintaining Momentum for Weight Loss and Muscle Building

In the first three weeks, the focus is on maintaining the momentum from the 28-Day Jumpstart. You'll continue to eat high-protein, low-carb meals that keep you feeling full and energized. The emphasis is on portion control, consistency, and gradually incorporating more variety into your diet. These weeks help you reinforce the habits you've built and sustain the progress you've made.

DAY	BREAKFAST	LUNCH	DINNER
Day 1	8. Oats with Almond Butter & Bananas	23. Spaghetti Squash with Meatballs	38. Garlic Parmesan Crusted Chicken
Day 2	9. Ham & Cheese Roll-Ups	24. Kale & Quinoa Salad	39. Creamy Tuscan Garlic Chicken
Day 3	10. Protein Pancakes	25. Tuna Avocado Sandwich	40. Cajun Chicken & Cauliflower Rice

Day 4	11. Burritos	26. Spicy Shrimp Lettuce Wraps	41. Chicken Sausage & Peppers
Day 5	12. Sausage & Egg Skillet	27. Zucchini Noodles with Pesto & Chicken	42. Teriyaki Salmon
Day 6	13. Turkey Bacon & Egg Cups	28. Asian Chicken Salad	43. Coconut Curry Chicken
Day 7	14. Low-Carb Pizza	29. Eggplant & Hummus Wrap	44. Beef Fajita Bowls

DAY	BREAKFAST	LUNCH	DINNER
Day 8	15. Salmon & Asparagus Frittata	23. Spaghetti Squash with Meatballs	38. Garlic Parmesan Crusted Chicken
Day 9	16. Coconut Flour Waffles	24. Kale & Quinoa Salad	39. Creamy Tuscan Garlic Chicken
Day 10	17. Almond Butter Protein Bars	25. Tuna Avocado Sandwich	40. Cajun Chicken & Cauliflower Rice
Day 11	8. Oats with Almond Butter & Bananas	26. Spicy Shrimp Lettuce Wraps	41. Chicken Sausage & Peppers
Day 12	9. Ham & Cheese Roll-Ups	27. Zucchini Noodles with Pesto & Chicken	42. Teriyaki Salmon
Day 13	10. Protein Pancakes	28. Asian Chicken Salad	43. Coconut Curry Chicken
Day 14	11. Burritos	29. Eggplant & Hummus Wrap	44. Beef Fajita Bowls

Weeks 4-6: Focus on Muscle Toning and Portion Control

As you enter the next three weeks, you'll start to refine your meal portions to align more closely with your specific goals. For those looking to lose weight, portion sizes will be slightly reduced, while those aiming to gain muscle will increase their protein intake. You'll continue to enjoy a variety of meals, ensuring that you stay motivated and satisfied while reaching your objectives.

DAY	BREAKFAST	LUNCH	DINNER

Day 15	8. Oats with Almond Butter & Bananas	23. Spaghetti Squash with Meatballs	38. Garlic Parmesan Crusted Chicken
Day 16	9. Ham & Cheese Roll-Ups	24. Kale & Quinoa Salad	39. Creamy Tuscan Garlic Chicken
Day 17	10. Protein Pancakes	25. Tuna Avocado Sandwich	40. Cajun Chicken & Cauliflower Rice
Day 18	11. Burritos	26. Spicy Shrimp Lettuce Wraps	41. Chicken Sausage & Peppers
Day 19	12. Sausage & Egg Skillet	27. Zucchini Noodles with Pesto & Chicken	42. Teriyaki Salmon
Day 20	13. Turkey Bacon & Egg Cups	28. Asian Chicken Salad	43. Coconut Curry Chicken
Day 21	14. Low-Carb Pizza	29. Eggplant & Hummus Wrap	44. Beef Fajita Bowls

Weeks 7-9: Maintenance and Long-Term Sustainability

By now, your body has adapted to a healthier, low-carb, high-protein lifestyle, and the final phase of the plan is all about maintenance. The focus is on balancing your meals to support long-term sustainability, ensuring that you can stick to this lifestyle for the foreseeable future. Whether you're still aiming for weight loss or working on building muscle, these final weeks will help you solidify your goals.

DAY	BREAKFAST	LUNCH	DINNER
Day 22	15. Salmon & Asparagus Frittata	23. Spaghetti Squash with Meatballs	38. Garlic Parmesan Crusted Chicken
Day 23	16. Coconut Flour Waffles	24. Kale & Quinoa Salad	39. Creamy Tuscan Garlic Chicken
Day 24	17. Almond Butter Protein Bars	25. Tuna Avocado Sandwich	40. Cajun Chicken & Cauliflower Rice
Day 25	8. Oats with Almond Butter & Bananas	26. Spicy Shrimp Lettuce Wraps	41. Chicken Sausage & Peppers
Day 26	9. Ham & Cheese Roll-Ups	27. Zucchini Noodles with Pesto & Chicken	42. Teriyaki Salmon

Day 27	10. Protein Pancakes	28. Asian Chicken Salad	43. Coconut Curry Chicken
Day 28	11. Burritos	29. Eggplant & Hummus Wrap	44. Beef Fajita Bowls

Tailoring the Plan for Weight Loss or Muscle Gain

This 60-day plan can be adapted based on your personal goals—whether you're aiming to lose weight, gain muscle, or simply maintain your current progress. Here's how to adjust the plan according to your needs:

- **For Weight Loss**: Focus on keeping portion sizes moderate, avoid snacking between meals, and choose the lower-calorie options provided in the plan. Stay consistent with your workouts and ensure you're drinking plenty of water.

- **For Muscle Gain**: Increase your intake of protein-rich foods by slightly increasing the portion sizes of protein in your meals. Pair your increased protein intake with resistance training to help build muscle mass.

By following these guidelines and sticking to the plan, you'll be able to reach your goals sustainably while still enjoying delicious, satisfying meals.

CHAPTER 10

How to Calculate and Adjust Your Caloric Needs

Understanding your caloric needs is essential to achieving your fitness goals, whether you're aiming for weight loss, muscle gain, or simply maintaining your current weight. Your daily caloric requirement is the number of calories your body needs to function effectively. This requirement is influenced by several factors, including your age, weight, height, activity level, and fitness goals. In this chapter, we'll walk you through how to calculate your caloric needs and adjust your intake as your body changes and progresses through the plan.

Once you've determined your caloric needs, you'll learn how to monitor your progress and adjust your meal plan to ensure continued success. Whether you're cutting calories for fat loss or increasing them for muscle growth, this chapter will provide a clear guide to navigating those changes.

Calculating Your Daily Caloric Requirements

The first step in adjusting your nutrition plan is understanding how many calories your body needs each day. This is known as your Total Daily Energy Expenditure (TDEE), which represents the number of calories you burn through basic bodily functions (your Basal Metabolic Rate, or BMR) plus physical activity.

Step 1: Calculate Your Basal Metabolic Rate (BMR)

Your **BMR** is the number of calories your body needs to maintain its basic functions, such as breathing, digestion, and circulation, while at rest. It accounts for about 60-75% of your total daily caloric expenditure.

The most commonly used formula to calculate BMR is the **Mifflin-St Jeor Equation**, which is as follows:

- **For women**: BMR = 10 × weight (kg) + 6.25 × height (cm) − 5 × age (years) − 161
- **For men**: BMR = 10 × weight (kg) + 6.25 × height (cm) − 5 × age (years) + 5

Example Calculation:

Let's calculate the BMR for a 35-year-old woman who weighs 70 kg and is 165 cm tall:

- BMR = 10 × 70 + 6.25 × 165 − 5 × 35 − 161
- BMR = 700 + 1,031.25 − 175 − 161
- BMR ≈ 1,395 calories/day

This means that to maintain her body's basic functions, she needs approximately 1,395 calories each day.

Step 2: Calculate Your Total Daily Energy Expenditure (TDEE)

Once you know your BMR, you can calculate your **TDEE** by factoring in your activity level. This provides an estimate of how many calories you need each day based on your lifestyle and exercise habits.

To calculate TDEE, multiply your BMR by an activity factor that corresponds to your level of daily physical activity:

- **Sedentary** (little to no exercise): BMR × 1.2
- **Lightly active** (light exercise/sports 1-3 days a week): BMR × 1.375
- **Moderately active** (moderate exercise/sports 3-5 days a week): BMR × 1.55
- **Very active** (hard exercise/sports 6-7 days a week): BMR × 1.725
- **Super active** (very hard exercise & physical job or training twice a day): BMR × 1.9

Example Calculation:

Using the same woman's BMR of 1,395 calories, if she is moderately active (exercising 3-5 days a week), her TDEE would be:

- TDEE = 1,395 × 1.55
- TDEE ≈ 2,162 calories/day

This means she needs around 2,162 calories per day to maintain her current weight.

Adjusting Your Caloric Intake for Your Goals

Once you've calculated your TDEE, the next step is to adjust your caloric intake to align with your specific goals, whether it's weight loss, muscle gain, or weight maintenance.

For Weight Loss:

To lose weight, you'll need to consume fewer calories than your TDEE, creating a calorie deficit. A typical calorie deficit for weight loss is between **300-500 calories per day**. This will lead to a steady weight loss of about 0.5 to 1 kg (1 to 2 pounds) per week, which is considered a healthy and sustainable rate of fat loss.

- **Mild Calorie Deficit (300-500 calories)**: If your TDEE is 2,162 calories, aim for a daily intake of 1,662 to 1,862 calories to achieve weight loss.

For Muscle Gain:

If your goal is to build muscle, you'll need to consume more calories than your TDEE, creating a calorie surplus. To gain muscle without excess fat, you should aim to consume **200-300 calories above your TDEE**. Combine this with strength training to ensure the extra calories contribute to muscle growth rather than fat gain.

- **Mild Calorie Surplus (200-300 calories)**: If your TDEE is 2,162 calories, aim for a daily intake of 2,362 to 2,462 calories to gain muscle gradually.

For Weight Maintenance:

To maintain your weight, simply aim to consume around your TDEE each day. This ensures your calorie intake balances out with the calories you burn through daily activities and exercise.

Tracking Progress and Adjusting the Plan for Maximum Results

It's essential to track your progress over time to see how your body responds to your caloric intake and adjust accordingly. Here's how to monitor and adjust based on your results:

Step 1: Measure Progress Weekly

Track your weight and body measurements (such as waist, hips, and thighs) weekly. This will give you a clearer picture of whether you're losing fat, gaining muscle, or maintaining your weight. Additionally, pay attention to how your clothes fit and how you feel in terms of energy and strength.

- **For weight loss**, look for a gradual decrease of 0.5-1 kg (1-2 pounds) per week.
- **For muscle gain**, monitor for steady muscle growth without excessive fat gain (use body measurements and strength progress as indicators).

Step 2: Adjust Your Caloric Intake

If your progress stalls or you're not seeing the results you want, it may be time to adjust your caloric intake:

- **If weight loss stalls**, decrease your caloric intake by an additional 100-200 calories per day. However, avoid cutting too many calories, as this could slow your metabolism and make weight loss more challenging.

- **If muscle gain slows**, increase your caloric intake by an additional 100-200 calories per day, focusing on protein-rich foods that support muscle repair and growth.

Step 3: Monitor Energy Levels and Exercise Performance

Pay attention to how you feel during workouts and throughout the day. If you notice a lack of energy or declining performance in your strength training, it might be a sign that you're not eating enough to support your activity level. In such cases, slightly increasing your caloric intake can help.

Step 4: Use Apps and Tools to Track Your Intake

There are many apps and online tools available to help you track your caloric intake and macronutrients (proteins, fats, and carbohydrates). These can make it easier to stay within your target calorie range and ensure that you're eating the right balance of nutrients to support your goals.

Understanding and adjusting your caloric intake is a critical part of any fitness or weight management journey. By calculating your TDEE and aligning your nutrition plan with your goals, you're setting yourself up for success, whether you're aiming for weight loss, muscle gain, or simply maintaining a healthy, sustainable lifestyle.

By consistently tracking your progress and being flexible with your caloric needs, you'll be able to fine-tune your plan and continue making strides toward your ideal physique and optimal health. Empower yourself with the knowledge you've gained in this chapter and use it to take control of your body's unique needs, ensuring sustainable and long-lasting results.

CHAPTER 11

Easy Substitutions: Adapting Recipes to Fit Your Lifestyle

One of the greatest strengths of a low-carb, high-protein diet is its flexibility. Whether you're following a paleo, keto, gluten-free, or vegan lifestyle, there are plenty of easy substitutions that can adapt the recipes in this book to fit your personal needs and preferences. Whether you're cooking for yourself, a family with different dietary preferences, or accommodating allergies or intolerances, this chapter will guide you through making simple swaps to ensure that every recipe is suitable for your goals and tastes.

Paleo Substitutions

The paleo diet focuses on whole, unprocessed foods and eliminates grains, legumes, dairy, and processed sugars. Adapting the recipes in this book to fit a paleo lifestyle is quite simple with a few ingredient swaps.

Common Substitutions for Paleo Recipes:

- **Flours**: Use **almond flour**, **coconut flour**, or **cassava flour** instead of wheat or grain-based flours.
- **Sweeteners**: Replace any sugar or artificial sweeteners with **honey**, **maple syrup**, or **coconut sugar**.
- **Dairy**: Substitute dairy milk with **almond milk**, **coconut milk**, or **cashew milk**. Replace cream with **coconut cream**.
- **Grains**: Instead of rice or quinoa, use **cauliflower rice**, **zoodles** (zucchini noodles), or **spaghetti squash**.
- **Legumes**: Since legumes are excluded on paleo, replace beans and lentils with extra vegetables or **mushrooms** for added bulk.
- **Soy**: Swap out soy sauce for **coconut aminos**.

Example Paleo Substitutions:

- **Spaghetti Squash with Meatballs (Recipe 23)**: Replace any cheese with nutritional yeast and ensure the meatballs don't contain breadcrumbs. Use spaghetti squash in place of pasta.

- **Low-Carb Pizza (Recipe 14)**: Use a cauliflower crust and dairy-free cheese or simply eliminate the cheese, using extra vegetables for toppings.

Keto Substitutions

The keto diet is all about keeping carbs very low (usually under 50 grams per day) and increasing fats. While most of the recipes in this book are already low-carb, a few tweaks can make them keto-friendly.

Common Substitutions for Keto Recipes:

- **Sweeteners**: Replace sugar, honey, or maple syrup with **stevia, erythritol,** or **monk fruit** sweeteners, which are low-carb and keto-approved.
- **Fats**: Increase the healthy fats by adding more **avocado, olive oil, butter,** or **ghee** to your meals.
- **Vegetables**: Swap higher-carb vegetables (such as carrots or sweet potatoes) with **zucchini, spinach, broccoli,** or **cauliflower**.
- **Baking**: Use **almond flour** or **coconut flour** instead of wheat flour to keep recipes low-carb.

Example Keto Substitutions:

- **Scrambled Eggs with Spinach (Recipe 5)**: Add more butter or cream to increase the fat content, and make sure no milk is added to the eggs.
- **Pesto Zoodles with Chicken (Recipe 35)**: Add more olive oil or cheese to increase the fat content, and ensure the pesto sauce doesn't contain added sugars.

Gluten-Free Substitutions

Going gluten-free can be seamless with the right swaps. Many of the recipes in this book are naturally gluten-free, but for those that aren't, there are easy adjustments you can make.

Common Substitutions for Gluten-Free Recipes:

- **Flours**: Replace wheat flour with **almond flour, coconut flour,** or **gluten-free all-purpose flour**.
- **Breadcrumbs**: Use **ground flaxseed, almond meal,** or **gluten-free panko** instead of traditional breadcrumbs.
- **Pasta**: Replace pasta with **zoodles, spaghetti squash,** or **gluten-free pasta** (made from chickpeas, quinoa, or lentils).

- **Soy Sauce**: Replace soy sauce with **gluten-free tamari** or **coconut aminos**.

Example Gluten-Free Substitutions:

- **Turkey Avocado Wrap (Recipe 17)**: Use a gluten-free tortilla or wrap, or opt for a lettuce wrap.
- **Eggplant Lasagna (Recipe 19)**: Use gluten-free breadcrumbs (or omit them entirely), and replace any flour in the sauce with a gluten-free thickener like arrowroot powder or cornstarch.

Vegan Substitutions

Adapting recipes to fit a vegan lifestyle involves removing all animal products, including meat, dairy, and eggs. Fortunately, many plant-based substitutes are readily available.

Common Substitutions for Vegan Recipes:

- **Meat**: Replace meat with **tofu, tempeh, seitan**, or **legumes** like lentils and chickpeas.
- **Dairy**: Use **almond milk, coconut milk**, or **oat milk** instead of dairy milk. Replace cheese with **nutritional yeast** or vegan cheese.
- **Eggs**: Use **flax eggs** (1 tablespoon ground flaxseed + 3 tablespoons water) or **chia eggs** as a binder in recipes that call for eggs.
- **Protein**: Ensure you're getting enough protein by adding plant-based sources like **tofu, tempeh, lentils**, and **quinoa**.

Example Vegan Substitutions:

- **Greek Yogurt Parfait (Recipe 1)**: Replace the Greek yogurt with coconut or almond milk yogurt, and use agave syrup instead of honey.
- **Chicken & Vegetable Skewers (Recipe 22)**: Replace the chicken with marinated tofu or tempeh and ensure the marinade doesn't contain honey or animal products.

Simple Adjustments for Personal or Family Preferences

Whether you're cooking for picky eaters, adapting meals for kids, or accommodating allergies, simple adjustments can make a big difference without compromising flavor or nutrition. Here are a few common adjustments to consider:

For Kids:

- **Texture**: Kids often have texture preferences. Smooth out soups, sauces, and smoothies by blending them or cutting vegetables into small, manageable pieces.
- **Flavors**: For kids who prefer mild flavors, reduce spices or keep sauces on the side so they can adjust to their taste.
- **Sneaking in Veggies**: Incorporate vegetables into dishes where they may go unnoticed, like blending spinach into a smoothie or grating zucchini into muffins.

For Allergies:

- **Nut Allergies**: Replace almond butter or other nut-based ingredients with **sunflower seed butter** or **tahini**.
- **Dairy Allergies**: Use **coconut milk**, **almond milk**, or **oat milk** in place of cow's milk, and substitute cheese with vegan cheese options.
- **Egg Allergies**: Use **flax eggs** or **chia eggs** as a replacement in recipes that require eggs for binding.

Tailoring Recipes for Weight Loss or Muscle Gain

While this book focuses on a low-carb, high-protein diet, the calorie content of each recipe can be adjusted depending on your specific goals. Here's how to make simple changes for either weight loss or muscle gain:

For Weight Loss:

- **Portion Control**: Reduce portion sizes, especially for high-fat ingredients like cheese, nuts, and oils.
- **Lean Protein**: Focus on lean protein sources like chicken breast, turkey, and fish. Limit fattier cuts of meat like steak or pork.
- **Vegetable Fillers**: Add more low-carb vegetables (such as spinach, broccoli, and cauliflower) to meals to increase volume without adding extra calories.

For Muscle Gain:

- **Increase Protein**: Add extra portions of protein to each meal. For example, double the chicken breast in a recipe or add an extra scoop of protein powder to your smoothies.
- **Healthy Fats**: Increase healthy fats like avocado, olive oil, and nuts to support muscle growth and provide extra calories.
- **Carb Timing**: While carbs are generally limited, timing them around workouts can be

beneficial for muscle recovery. Consider adding sweet potatoes, quinoa, or other complex carbs to post-workout meals.

The key to sustaining a low-carb, high-protein lifestyle is flexibility. By making easy substitutions and adjustments, you can customize these recipes to meet your dietary needs, preferences, and goals. Whether you're following a paleo, keto, gluten-free, or vegan diet, or simply adjusting for allergies or family preferences, this chapter empowers you to adapt every meal to your unique lifestyle. The possibilities are endless, and with a little creativity, you can enjoy a wide variety of nutritious, delicious, and satisfying meals tailored to your needs.

PART 4

ADDITIONAL RESOURCES AND SUPPORT

CHAPTER 12

Staying Motivated: Tips and Success Stories

Embarking on a low-carb, high-protein lifestyle can feel exciting at first, especially when you start to experience the positive changes in your body and energy levels. However, as time goes on, maintaining that initial momentum can become challenging. Busy schedules, family obligations, and personal setbacks often threaten to derail progress, making it easy to slip back into old habits. Staying motivated is the key to long-term success, and fortunately, there are proven strategies that can help you stay focused on your goals, even when life gets hectic.

Motivation isn't just about willpower or self-discipline. It's about building a system of habits and routines that support your goals, surrounding yourself with a support network, and reminding yourself why you started this journey in the first place. Motivation is also deeply personal, and what works for one person may not work for another. That's why it's important to approach this lifestyle with flexibility and an open mind, willing to adapt as you go. In this chapter, we'll explore how to stay focused, remain consistent, and find inspiration through the stories of others who have made this lifestyle work for them, even in the busiest of circumstances.

How to Stay Focused and Consistent

Staying consistent with any new lifestyle requires intention and planning. It's easy to start strong, but without a solid foundation of habits, even the best intentions can fade. One of the best ways to remain focused is by setting clear and achievable goals. These goals act as your personal guideposts, helping you measure progress and giving you something concrete to work toward. Whether your goal is to lose weight, build muscle, or simply feel healthier, having specific targets can make all the difference. Many people find it helpful to break their goals down into smaller milestones, celebrating the small victories along the way. A drop in the number on the scale, fitting into an old pair of jeans, or lifting a heavier weight at the gym are all signs that your hard work is paying off.

But beyond the goals themselves, having a plan is crucial. A structured meal plan can take the guesswork out of everyday decisions. Preparing meals ahead of time ensures that when the busy workweek hits, you aren't tempted to grab something unhealthy just because it's convenient. Knowing exactly what you're going to eat and when you're going to exercise simplifies your daily routine, leaving less room for distractions or excuses. But even with the best-laid plans, obstacles are inevitable. Life doesn't always go according to schedule, and when disruptions arise, having a backup plan can help you stay on track. Whether it's keeping healthy snacks at your desk or scheduling a shorter, more intense workout when time is tight, flexibility is key to maintaining consistency.

A powerful tool in staying consistent is the support of others. The journey toward better health is often more successful when shared with others. Whether it's a workout partner, a meal-prep buddy, or a supportive online community, being accountable to someone can keep you motivated. It's not just about accountability, though—sharing your progress with others, celebrating successes, and even voicing your struggles can provide the encouragement needed to keep going. If you're surrounded by people who believe in your goals and want to see you succeed, it can make the journey much less lonely. Some people find support in fitness classes, while others turn to online groups where like-minded individuals share recipes, workout routines, and motivation. The important thing is finding what works for you and leaning on that support system when you need it most.

Staying motivated is about more than just seeing progress on the scale or in the mirror. There will be times when the numbers don't move, and it's in these moments that you need to focus on non-scale victories. These are the smaller but equally important signs of progress, like waking up feeling more energized, noticing that your clothes fit better, or realizing that you no longer crave unhealthy foods. These moments are often overlooked but serve as powerful reminders that the effort you're putting in is making a difference. Weight isn't the only measure of success, and focusing solely on the scale can sometimes lead to frustration. By broadening your perspective, you can stay motivated even when the numbers aren't moving as fast as you'd like.

Of course, it's essential to cultivate a mindset that's positive and flexible. Challenges are inevitable, but setbacks don't have to mean failure. It's natural to have days where you indulge in something outside of your plan or skip a workout. What matters most is how you respond to these moments. Instead of feeling guilty or discouraged, view them as learning experiences and move forward with renewed focus. Maintaining a balanced mindset allows you to adjust your approach as needed without feeling like you've "ruined" your progress. Flexibility is key to long-term success because life will always throw curveballs, but how you handle them determines whether you stay on track or give up entirely.

Inspiring Stories of Busy People Who Made It Work

When the going gets tough, it can be incredibly helpful to draw inspiration from those who have walked the same path. Real-life stories of individuals who have successfully adopted and maintained a low-carb, high-protein lifestyle despite their hectic lives show us that it is possible to prioritize health, even when it feels like there's no time. These stories demonstrate that with the right mindset and strategies, you can balance work, family, and personal health goals.

Take Emily, for example. A 35-year-old marketing manager and mother of two, Emily's life is a whirlwind of work deadlines, school pickups, and family dinners. For years, she struggled to find the time and energy to focus on her own health. Between managing her career and caring for her children, it felt impossible to make time for healthy meals and regular exercise. However, after reaching a point of frustration with her energy levels and weight, Emily decided it was time for a change. She started small, carving out time every Sunday to prep meals for the week ahead. This one habit became her saving grace. By having healthy meals ready to go, she avoided the temptation of grabbing takeout during busy weekdays. Within three months, Emily had lost 15 pounds, felt more energetic, and noticed significant improvements in her fitness levels. Her advice: "Meal prepping gave me control over my health in a way that didn't feel overwhelming. It was the one thing I could do for myself in the midst of all my responsibilities."

Carlos, a 42-year-old corporate executive, also faced challenges maintaining a healthy lifestyle while managing a demanding job that required frequent travel. Long hours and business dinners made it difficult for him to stick to a regular routine, and after noticing his weight creeping up, he knew something had to change. Carlos started by making small adjustments—choosing healthier options at restaurants, packing protein bars for flights, and finding time for quick hotel room workouts. Over the course of six months, he lost 25 pounds and drastically improved his energy levels. What made the difference for Carlos was realizing that he didn't need to be perfect; he just needed to make smarter choices consistently. "I learned that it wasn't about being perfect every day. It was about making more good decisions than bad ones, and over time, those small decisions added up."

Jasmine, a 23-year-old nursing student, had her own struggles with staying healthy amid a packed schedule of classes, clinical rotations, and a part-time job. Always on the go, Jasmine relied on fast food to get her through the day, leaving her feeling sluggish and unmotivated. After researching low-carb, high-protein diets, she decided to give it a try. Jasmine began packing her lunches and snacks to avoid the temptation of grabbing something unhealthy on campus. She found that by planning her meals the night before and keeping healthy snacks in her bag, she was able to make better choices throughout the day. The results were transformative—not only did she lose weight, but she also felt more energized and focused during her long days of study and clinical work. "I never thought I could find the time to prioritize my health while in school, but once I started planning ahead, it became second nature."

These stories are just a few examples of how everyday people with busy lives have made the low-carb, high-protein lifestyle work for them. Their successes didn't come from perfection but from consistency, planning, and a willingness to adapt. They remind us that even in the busiest of lives, there's always room to prioritize health. If they can do it, so can you.

New version of GPT available - Continue chatting to use the old version, or start a new chat for the latest version.

CONCLUSION
Your Journey to a Healthier, Stronger You

Embarking on a low-carb, high-protein lifestyle is more than just a dietary change; it's a complete shift in how you approach your health, wellness, and everyday life. Over the course of this book, we've covered everything from the science behind this eating plan to meal prep strategies, delicious recipes, and tips for staying motivated. But now, as we reach the conclusion, it's important to reflect on the journey you've taken and to prepare yourself for the road ahead.

The low-carb, high-protein lifestyle isn't just a short-term fix or a quick way to shed a few pounds. It's a sustainable, long-term approach to nutrition that helps you build a foundation for a healthier life. As you've learned, this way of eating helps regulate your energy levels, control hunger, support weight loss, build muscle, and improve overall health. The beauty of this lifestyle is that it's adaptable—it can fit into any schedule, work for various dietary needs, and can be modified for specific fitness goals like weight loss or muscle gain.

One of the most important lessons to take away from this journey is that every step you take toward better health matters. Whether you've already reached your initial goals or are still working toward them, the progress you've made is worth celebrating. Healthy living is a marathon, not a sprint, and the most successful people are those who embrace the ups and downs along the way, using setbacks as learning opportunities rather than reasons to give up.

As you move forward, one of your biggest assets will be the habits you've developed along the way. Building habits that support your health goals is crucial to maintaining your progress. This might include meal prepping on Sundays, choosing healthier options when eating out, or making time for regular exercise. Whatever your routines are, the key to long-term success lies in consistency. The more ingrained these habits become, the easier they will be to maintain over the long haul, even when life gets busy.

If you haven't already developed these habits, don't worry. Start small, and focus on one change at a time. Begin with something manageable, like drinking more water each day or preparing your lunch the night before. Once that habit becomes part of your routine, add another small change. Over time, these small changes will add up to significant improvements in your health.

Another essential aspect of maintaining long-term success is flexibility. Life is full of unexpected changes—whether it's a busy workweek, a vacation, or a family emergency, there will be times when your routine is disrupted. The key is to adapt without letting setbacks derail your progress entirely. If you have a week where you can't stick to your plan perfectly, remember that it's okay. Simply pick up where you left off as soon as you can. Flexibility allows you to stay on track without becoming overwhelmed by the pressure to be perfect all the time.

One of the most empowering aspects of this lifestyle is learning to listen to your body. As you've likely experienced, a low-carb, high-protein diet naturally helps you tune into your hunger and fullness cues. When you eat protein-rich meals, you feel full and satisfied for longer, which can help you avoid overeating. Paying attention to how your body responds to different foods, workouts, and sleep patterns is key to staying healthy in the long run.

As you continue on this journey, don't be afraid to adjust your diet based on what your body is telling you. If you find that certain foods aren't working for you anymore, or that your energy levels are dipping, take the time to reassess and make changes. Your body's needs can evolve over time, especially as you hit new fitness milestones or enter different stages of life.

Motivation will always be a critical component of your success. There will be days when you feel incredibly motivated to stick to your plan, and other days when it feels like a struggle. What's important is to recognize that motivation ebbs and flows, and to have strategies in place to keep yourself moving forward, even when the going gets tough.

One of the best ways to stay motivated is to remind yourself of why you started. Reconnect with the reasons behind your goals, whether it's to improve your health, feel more energetic, lose weight, or build muscle. Reflect on how far you've come and the progress you've made, both in terms of physical changes and how you feel mentally and emotionally.

Another key strategy is to surround yourself with support. Whether it's friends, family, or an online community, having people who encourage and support you can make all the difference. Share your journey with them—your wins, your struggles, and everything in between. They can provide valuable encouragement on days when your motivation is low, and celebrating your successes with others makes the journey more rewarding.

One of the greatest strengths of the low-carb, high-protein lifestyle is its adaptability. As you continue to pursue your health and fitness goals, you can tailor your eating plan to fit your needs. Whether you want to focus on muscle gain, fat loss, or simply maintaining your current health, this approach is flexible enough to support your goals.

If, for example, you find that your goals shift over time—from losing weight to maintaining it, or from focusing on health to building more muscle—you can make small adjustments to your diet and workout routine to align with those new priorities. This lifestyle doesn't require rigid rules, and that flexibility allows it to grow and evolve with you.

Additionally, this approach is family-friendly and can be adapted to different dietary preferences. Whether you're cooking for yourself, a partner, or your children, the recipes and meal plans in this book can be modified to fit everyone's tastes and needs. This makes it easier to maintain the lifestyle without feeling like you have to prepare separate meals for yourself and your family.

Now that you've learned the ins and outs of a low-carb, high-protein lifestyle, you're well-equipped to continue on your journey with confidence. You've mastered the basics, developed healthy habits, and found motivation through success stories and practical tips. The future is bright, and with each new day, you have the opportunity to continue improving your health, building strength, and becoming the best version of yourself.

As you move forward, remember that this journey is uniquely yours. Celebrate your successes, no matter how small, and don't be discouraged by setbacks. The path to better health is filled with learning opportunities, and each step you take brings you closer to your goals. Trust the process, believe in your ability to succeed, and keep moving forward.

The tools, strategies, and knowledge you've gained throughout this book will serve you well as you continue on your low-carb, high-protein journey. Whether you're focused on maintaining your progress, pushing yourself to new fitness goals, or simply enjoying the benefits of a healthier, more vibrant life, you have everything you need to succeed.

Here's to a healthier, stronger, and more confident you. Keep going—you've got this.

Index of Recipes

Made in the USA
Middletown, DE
15 December 2024

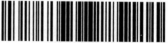